YOUR GUT FEELINGS

YOUR GUT FEELINGS

A Complete Guide to
Living Better
with Intestinal Problems

Henry D. Janowitz, M.D.

New York   Oxford
OXFORD UNIVERSITY PRESS
1987

Oxford University Press

Oxford   New York   Toronto
Delhi   Bombay   Calcutta   Madras   Karachi
Petaling Jaya   Singapore   Hong Kong   Tokyo
Nairobi   Dar es Salaam   Cape Town
Melbourne   Auckland

and associated companies in
Beirut   Berlin   Ibadan   Nicosia

Copyright © 1987 by Henry D. Janowitz

Published by Oxford University Press, Inc.,
200 Madison Avenue, New York, New York 10016

Oxford is a registered trademark of Oxford University Press

Library of Congress Cataloging-in-Publication Data
Janowitz, Henry D.
Your gut feelings.
Bibliography: p.   1. Intestines—Diseases—Popular works.
I. Title. RC860.J33   1987   616.3'4   87-7679
ISBN 0-19-504309-X

1 3 5 7 9 8 6 4 2

Printed in the United States of America
on acid-free paper

For Addy, Annie, and Mary

Preface

The subtitle of this book might well have been *A guide for those perplexed about their bowels*. It is not designed to be a textbook of medicine for the layperson, but to inform him or her about the common disorders of the lower intestinal tract and to offer ways of coping with them and approaches to prevention.

Not only scientific advances, but until recently even accepted information about this area of the body, have lagged behind the rest of modern medicine. We are finally, leaving behind the vestiges of Victorian prudery. Presidents have shown their abdominal scars to the public, and everyone knows about President Reagan's colonoscopy. The general public is anxious for information, but this area has been relatively neglected. In the field of gastrointestinal function, disturbances and diseases, there have been popular books on gall stones, peptic ulcers, and nervous indigestion, but few on the bowel and its activities. One aim of this book is to remedy this deficiency.

Now that methods for studying and treating the human colon are advancing rapidly, a second aim of this book is to present these newer methods and instruments in the proper perspective, especially the risks that they carry. Someone undergoing a test should understand why it is being done, its advantages and disadvantages, and how it will help to decide his or her future treatment. In our age of consumerism these decisions are joint ones, and informed consent requires a very well-informed patient in addition to a well-informed doctor.

I also hope that this book will help readers decide whether or not to pursue some of the day-to-day signals they may get from their intestinal tracts. Belly aches, gas rumbling, diarrhea, constipation, and rectal bleeding are relatively common experiences. We all need some guidelines. These frequent occurrences need not have serious consequences but some patterns need prompt attention.

These disorders deserve our attention because of their widespread incidence, their cost in loss of income due to absenteeism, and their toll in pain and suffering. *The irritable bowel syndrome* (IBS) is the commonest reason why people consult gastroenterologists and probably among the commonest reasons why they go to doctors in general and are admitted to hospitals. Since this if often a diagnosis of exclusion, it is of utmost importance that the patient understand the aim of investigation. The intent of the section on IBS is to help him or her participate and cooperate in the diagnosis, and to set the stage for that necessary review of dietary habits and life styles which are now considered essential if the condition is to be managed successfully and prevented in the future.

Inflammatory bowel disease (IBD) remains the most baffling of the intestinal disorders despite fifty years of intense research. The management of these disorders, which strike young people at critical times in their development—when education is being completed or a career launched—requires not only the cooperation but the understanding of parents, spouses, and siblings for the best care of the afflicted individual.

Diarrhea, constipation, "gas," and rectal bleeding are common problems requiring varying degrees of study to "cure" and to prevent their recurrence.

Colo-rectal cancer is steadily increasing in the United States and will claim 60,000 lives next year. The prevention of this disease requires understanding the possible role of diet, monitoring rectal bleeding, and searching for and removing *polyps* of the colon which are the precursors of these cancers.

Americans, like the rest of the Western world, are preoccupied with diets and dieting and the quest for "healthy" foods. The chapter on *"food allergies:* fact and/or fiction" addresses the question of food intolerances, with a practical approach to their management.

In a world in which the population is growing older, in an age when the aged are being separated into the "young-old" and the "old-old," it is appropriate that we should consider the *aging gut.* In a society of sexual permissiveness we also need to have a brief acquaintanceship with the *sexually transmitted bowel diseases* (STBD).

Our intestinal tract is not floating free in outer space; disturbances in other parts of our bodies, in other organ systems, have their intestinal repercussions. A frequently overlooked area is the effect of modern drugs and medicines on the functioning of the lower bowel. Both of these merit discussion.

This volume concludes with a discussion of the possible role of emotions on the functioning of the intestine and their effects on diseases of the bowel—what I call the *"brain-gut connection."*

If this book guides without being dictatorial, enlightens without overwhelming its readers with facts, informs without frightening, and encourages a cooperative dialogue between patient and doctor, then it will have accomplished its author's intent. I have not wanted to make part-time doctors out of its readers, but to encourage the development of that informed, medically literate public modern medicine needs in this complex technological age.

New York   H. D. J.
January 1987

Acknowledgments

This book owes most to my patients with gastrointestinal complaints. Their pointed questions, especially those of the "worried well," have helped me to communicate better with them.

Dr. Jerome Waye obtained the photographs of the colonic diagnostic instruments and especially the endoscopic pictures. Dr. Daniel Maklansky prepared the radiographs. Dr. Samuel Meyers read the manuscript carefully and also supplied me with endoscopic photographs.

The entire manuscript has profited greatly from the rigorous yet sympathetic care of my editor, Shelley Reinhardt, to whom I am happy to give these thanks.

Contents

1 The Lower Intestinal Tract
  An Overview   3
2 The Irritable Bowel Syndrome (IBS)   14
3 Inflammatory Bowel Diseases
  The Serious Inflammations   35
    Finding out what's wrong   35
    Once the diagnosis of IBD is made   50
    Frequently asked questions about IBD   68
4 Diarrhea, Constipation, and Rectal Bleeding   78
5 Polyps and Cancer of the Colon
  Prevention and Treatment of Cancer of the
  Colon   112
6 Diverticula, Diverticulosis and Diverticulitis
  Pockets and Boils   133
7 Food Allergies Fact and/or Fancy   146
8 The Aging Gut   156
9 Intestinal Repercussions of Other Diseases   165

10 Medicines and the Gut   *169*
11 Intestinal Gas
    What is it? What does it come from? What can
    we do about it?   *177*
12 Sexually Transmitted Bowel Diseases (STBD)   *181*
13 The Abdominal Pain Without a Name   *185*
14 Your Gut Feelings
    The Brain-Gut Connection   *187*

    Suggested Reading   *195*

    Index   *197*

YOUR GUT FEELINGS

1

The Lower Intestinal Tract

An Overview

This book focuses on disturbances of the lower intestinal tract or "the gut." However, it is important to realize that the entire gastrointestinal tract is a wonderfully coordinated and programmed apparatus for our entire nutritional intake, its transportation and mechanical "blenderizing," the digestion and absorption of the essential, vital materials and, finally, the storage of the waste residues and their periodic evacuation. The lower intestinal tract is a part of this machinery and must do its work at the correct time to insure harmonious, coordinated functioning.

The gastrointestinal tract, which reaches from your mouth, passes through the chest, occupies the bulk of the abdomen, and ends in the rectum, accomplishes this complicated task with the help of secretions from adjoining glands: the salivary glands in the mouth, and the liver and pancreas in the abdominal cavity. The salivary glands secrete saliva, which begins the breakdown of food. The liver secretes bile, important in the digestion of fats, which is stored in the gallbladder. The pancreas simultaneously pours forth

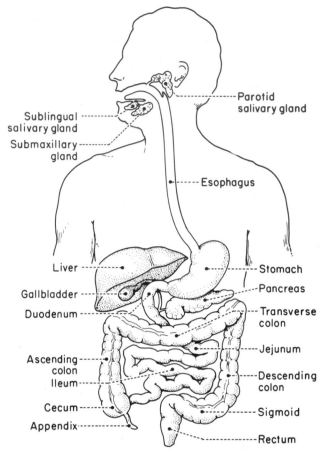

FIGURE 1.1 Diagram of the gastrointestinal tract from mouth to rectum.

its juices containing the digestive enzymes, which split fats, sugars, and protein.

It will help to visualize this long tube, a veritable hydraulic system moving solids and liquids along, by looking at Figure 1.1. In the mouth, the tongue and teeth help to get digestion started by chewing and breaking down our foods into smaller pieces. The three groups of *salivary glands* help by moistening these pieces, thus allowing us to taste and enjoy the process; they also secrete the digestive enzymes amylase and lipase, which help digest starch and fat.

Swallowing is a very complicated, coordinated act that starts out under our control as food is pushed into the back of our throats. This is followed by the automatic opening of the gate at the upper end of the esophagus, whose sole job is to move the swallowed materials through the chest to the stomach. A valve at the lower end of the esophagus, the lower esophageal spincter, opens normally as the peristaltic contractions of the esophagus sweep its contents down.

In the stomach, digestion is continued mainly by the process of mechanically grinding the swallowed foods, liquefied by the *acid* that the stomach pours out, aided by the enzyme *pepsin,* which begins to digest the protein of our foods.

The contractions of the stomach, having reduced the materials into manageable smaller particles, then progressively empty the stomach and move its contents into the long, narrow *small intestine.* It is here that the major part of digestion and absorption takes place. In the first part of the small intestine, known as the *duodenum,* bile and pancreative juice are added to the digestive mixture. In the second portion, the *jejunum,* fats, starches, and proteins arc broken down to their smallest components and absorbed by the lining cells of the bowel, as the contents are being moved along as on a conveyor belt. In the third or lowest portion of the small bowel, the *ileum,* water is absorbed, along with calcium, other minerals, and vitamins (especially vitamin B_{12}); and bile is recaptured and reabsorbed to prevent its loss from the body.

Large amounts of water have been pumped into the small intestine in the course of the digestive process: swallowed saliva, the water we drink, the acidic fluid secreted by the stomach, bile and pancreatic juice, as well as fluid secreted by the upper small bowel itself—in all perhaps up to 8–10 quarts. Most of this, however, will be put back nicely into the body by the lining cells that pump this large amount of fluid back.

By this time, the undigested food residuals and perhaps about 1 quart of fluid leave the ileum and enter the right side of the *colon* (Figure 1.2). Here this loose watery mixture is dehydrated and compacted by the *cecum* and *ascending colon* and temporarily stored in the *transverse colon*. Once or twice a day the more solid contents of the colon are moved into the *descending colon* and *rectosigmoid colon* by what is called a mass peristaltic movement.

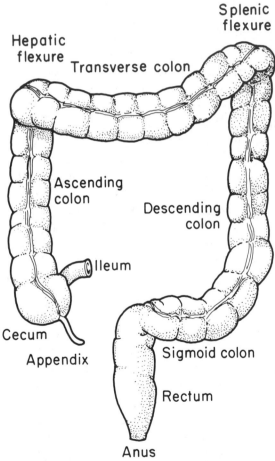

FIGURE 1.2 Diagram of the colon (the large bowel).

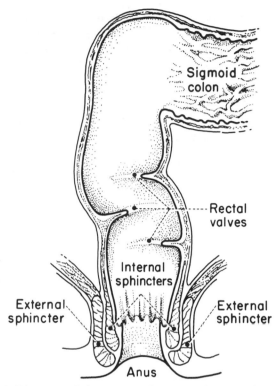

FIGURE 1.3 Diagram of the anus and rectum showing the internal and external sphincters, the muscular valves involved in defecation.

The presence of this mass of stool in the rectum gives rise to the sensations we recognize as the need to move our bowels. The gatekeepers at the lower end of the rectum and anus, the *internal and external rectal sphincters* (Figure 1.3), respond appropriately and the rectal contents are evacuated, again in a well-coordinated action under our voluntary control in the normal healthy state.

Although we will be concerned here mainly with what goes on and what may go wrong with the small intestine and colon—-referred to collectively as the *bowels*—you can see that disturbances at points upstream can lead to disturbances downstream.

The striking thing about the intestinal tract is that from below the mouth up to the colon, the entire intestine is relatively sterile and few bacteria live there. The acid of the stomach is believed to act like a disinfectant and prevent the growth of organisms, harmless ones as well as dangerous kinds. The human colon, however, contains an amazing variety of bacterial organisms. There are at least 400 distinct species, although 15 types account for the majority of them. About one-third of the material in the colon is bacterial, and at least half of the stool is also made up of bacteria. So you can see that even when starving or not eating any food, you can still have bowel movements, although the number and size of the feces are reduced considerably. Earlier in the century, "professional starvers" used to travel with sideshows and circuses. When they were studied in scientific laboratories, it was learned that they continued to have bowel movements.

Intestinal Sensations

It is difficult to put into words the kinds of discomfort we experience in the abdomen, the entire area below the chest, from the diaphragm to the groin. Further, these sensations are private. No one else experiences our feelings. Yet we all must talk about our sensations, including pains, if we are to make sense to our doctors and help them to give us relief.

This is not a textbook of medicine or of the nervous system, but it is important to realize that the study of pains still remains a mysterious business. No matter where you feel them, sensations that arise anywhere in the body are carried to the spinal cord and to localized areas in the brain, where they are perceived by the rich sets of nerves our bodies and organs are supplied with. Some supply information to the central nervous system from the exterior. In the case of the surface of the abdomen, these are called *cutaneous* or *somatic* nerves. Another set of nerves carries impulses from deep within the body. The nerves that carry sensation from our gastrointestinal tract, or the viscera, are called the *visceral nerve sets*.

While the skin can sense a number of feelings: hot, cold, touch, itch, tickle, location, and pain, the intestinal tract really can feel only pain. Further, the two sets, cutaneous and visceral nerves, are so connected that pain coming from the intestine or its associated glands (liver and pancreas) is often "referred" to certain locations on the skin. *Referred pain* is felt in addition to the pain that arises in the intestinal organs themselves, the so-called *true visceral pain* (see Figure 1.4 for referred pain).

Pain we feel on the skin can be set off by a variety of stimuli, such as excess heat, cold, or pressure. In contrast, the intestinal tract can perceive only a few things. The gut can be cut, for instance, without our feeling very much of anything. The thing that sets off pain signals from our gut is the stretching or pulling or swelling or expansion of the muscles of the bowel wall. When this occurs, we feel pain from our intestine.

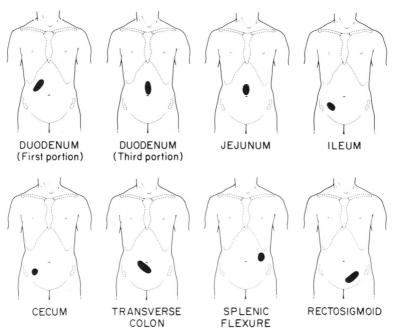

DUODENUM (First portion)   DUODENUM (Third portion)   JEJUNUM   ILEUM

CECUM   TRANSVERSE COLON   SPLENIC FLEXURE   RECTOSIGMOID

FIGURE 1.4 Diagram indicating the places on the abdominal skin where "referred pain" that arises in the intestinal tract may be felt.

As the intestine moves its contents along by the peristaltic contractions of the intestinal wall muscles, we usually feel no sensation. Occasionally one can hear splashes or gurgles as the intestine pushes mixtures of air and fluid contents along. Unless we have some disease or inflammation, swallowing gives rise to no sensations as food moves down the esophagus. When the stomach is empty or emptying itself, it contracts rhythmically at times, and sometimes these contractions can be heard. We speak of our stomachs as "talking," or "growling." When we are hungry, and the contractions of the stomach become stronger and stronger, we feel "hunger pangs," mainly in the upper abdomen, usually a little to the left of the midline.

The intestines normally do not give rise to any painful or uncomfortable sensations as they move material along the entire tract from the small bowel into the colon. As the contents of the right side of the colon move into the left side and the rectum is filled with stool, this distends the rectal area and gives rise to the sensation of needing to defecate and empty the rectum.

Pain arises when contractions of the intestine increase in intensity from the peristaltic muscle movements. Since these contractions occur in a rhythmic regular pattern of contraction and relaxation, we experience pain or discomfort of a periodic or rhythmic nature. These sensations grab us, then relax, then recur again and again. It is this kind of pain that gives us stomach or abdominal "cramps," similar to the contractions of the uterus in labor. When the contractions of the intestine muscles are sustained without periods of relaxation, they give rise to the feeling we recognize as a "spasm."

It is often difficult to realize that a pain can be caused by simple contractions of the intestines. Yet if you make a fist and hold your hand closed for 5 minutes, it hurts. If you hold your hand tightly closed for 25 minutes, you will have a very sore hand. The same kind of severe pain can be caused by sustained contractions of the gut without relaxation.

At this point I want to emphasize that all the movements along the intestine I have been describing take place because the gut actually is a continuous muscular tube. It is made up of two sets of muscles, one circular, which surrounds the inner lining, and one longitudinal, which runs lengthwise outside the inner circular layer. Their coordinated contractions move materials along the "conveyor belt" I have called the gut. Many of the sensations from the intestines that give us discomfort result from disturbances in the movement or motility of this long water-and-gas-containing tube. Most of those that are not caused by diseases of the intestine are now considered to have their basis in disorders of motility.

In both the small intestine and the colon, the cells of the muscle layers (the longitudinal ones in the intestine and the circular ones in the colon) generate electrical signals that pace and regulate the rhythmical contractions. These electrical impulses coordinate the activities of adjacent cells over long distances in the intestine. The nerves from the brain and spinal cord in turn influence the automatic action of the intestinal muscle cells and layers. One can thus visualize how disturbances in the electrical or nervous impulses of the intestine could lead to disturbances in contractions and movements in the gut, and then to uncomfortable sensations.

The Location of Pain

Where you feel the pain can be an important clue to what is causing it. Pains we feel in the abdomen usually come from difficulties within the abdomen, but not always. For example, pain due to stones passing along the ducts from the kidneys to the bladder can start in the back or flanks of the body and extend down the right or left side of the front of the abdomen. Pain coming from problems of the lower half of the spine can move around to the front of the abdomen. They can *radiate* (as physicians call it) from where they start to another part of the body, because the nerves that carry the pain signals pass through that other area.

Some pains are felt directly in the portion of the abdomen where the offending organ lies. To locate and name the area, the front surface of the abdomen is divided into four quarters, or *quadrants* (Figure 1.5), labeled right or left, upper or lower. Pains in the liver and gallbladder usually are felt in the right upper quadrant, pain in

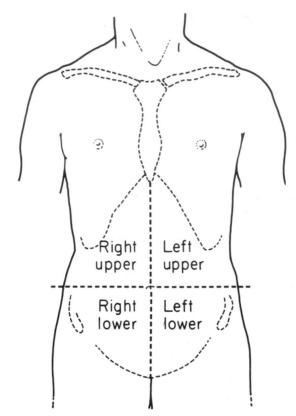

FIGURE 1.5 Schematic drawing of the abdomen, naming the four quadrants.

the stomach in the middle of the upper quadrants, close to the lower edge of the ribs. Another pain, which I call an "upstairs" pain, arises from the pancreas, which lies deep in the upper quadrants also in the midline. This pain is usually felt as a deep pain, deep, that is, inside, in contrast to the gallbladder or stomach pains that seem to be closer to the surface of the abdomen.

The pain and discomfort we are most concerned about in this book come from the small intestine and colon, which occupy the bulk of the space in the abdomen. It may be spread all over the place and can be felt in many areas.

Pain that comes from the colon, which is ordinarily tightly anchored in place, is most often felt in both lower quarters of the abdomen, low down and well below the belly button (the umbilicus). This is a "downstairs" pain in contrast to the "upper story" one of the stomach, pancreas, liver, and gallbladder. Yet, as you can see from the diagram, the colon lies in all four parts of the abdomen. So the correspondence of the organ with its pain pattern is not exact. Pain in the appendix, while it may start elsewhere, quickly moves to its exact anatomical location in the right lower quadrant. Pains arising from the sigmoid colon (Figure 1.2) are usually felt on the other side of the abdomen, in the left lower segment. It is here that the typical pains of diverticulitis are experienced.

The long small intestine is less closely tied down by its attachments, so its pains are felt all over the abdomen, but most typically in the middle area of all four quadrants and usually centering around the umbilicus.

2

The Irritable Bowel Syndrome (IBS)

How Do I Know I Have IBS?

You are a relatively young person, in your twenties, thirties, or forties, who enjoys good health. Without any warning you begin to experience periods of lower abdominal discomfort, which may increase in intensity. You have pain that feels like cramps. You need to move your bowels more often than usual and to move them quickly: "Precipitously" is your doctor's word for this urgent need. Suddenly your stools are different: loose, watery, even explosive, without blood but possibly containing mucus that looks like the uncooked white of an egg or the stuff you blow out of your nose with a simple cold.

This kind of disturbance in your intestine may repeat itself so that you begin to see a pattern. It happened before when you were a teenager, most inconveniently, just before taking an examination in high school or before going out on your first date. Or these periodic storms may be followed by times when your abdomen feels and even looks blown up; you feel distended, full of gas. The cramps return, but now you want to move your bowels and cannot.

The whole experience sounds a bit like what you have heard others talk about: the "nervous stomach." If you consult your doctor after it happens a few times, he or she reassuringly tells you that you are suffering from the *irritable bowel syndrome* (IBS).

You are a bit reassured when the doctor informs you after doing some tests that he or she cannot find any organic basis for the distress, but you are not much consoled when you learn that your condition is quite common; it helps only a little to know that many others are in the same boat. Perhaps 15% of the adult population has the same condition, although many never go to a doctor about it. Even so, the IBS is the commonest reason why patients in the United States consult gastroenterologists, the physicians who specialize in disorders of the gastrointestinal tract. However, statistics do not make one feel any better. I know a lot of people will lose their umbrellas in Grand Central Station, but I want to know about my umbrella. What is making my bowel so irritable?

This combination of symptoms and the change in the behavior of your lower intestinal tract, which physicians label the *irritable bowel syndrome* (a syndrome is just the name for a constellation of signs and symptoms that go together), has a multitude of names: the irritable bowel, the nervous gut, the unstable bowel, the adaptive colon, the spastic colon, the spastic bowel, among others. These terms are one way of labeling for convenience the group of symptoms that is bothering you. Although these diagnostic labels are not misleading, some other loosely used terms are. For a long time, when emphasis was placed on the passage of mucus with the bowel movements, the condition was called mucous colitis, and even now the IBS is called spastic colitis or just colitis. Unfortunately, this implies that the condition is an inflammation of the intestine and colon. This is not the case: There is no evidence that any inflammation is going on. It may lead you to think you are suffering from one of the more serious conditions (ulcerative colitis and Crohn's disease), which are discussed elsewhere in this book, and your concern about that may make you even more anxious about your condition and contribute to your discomfort.

You should know right away that no physician believes that the irritable bowel is a forerunner of ulcerative colitis or Crohn's disease, the so-called *inflammatory bowel diseases* (IBD), nor does the IBS become an inflammatory condition. It should also be stressed that IBS has nothing to do with the development of cancer of the colon. (Cancer of the small bowel or small intestine is one of the rarest diseases on earth.) As for the colon, the IBS is not a forerunner of either malignant tumors or the serious inflammation of ulcerative colitis and/or Crohn's disease.

Yet IBS can be very uncomfortable, and at times you may very well wonder and worry whether the hard, crampy abdominal discomfort you have can really be due to a nonorganic cause.

Is IBS a Wastebasket Diagnosis of All the Lower Bowel Disturbances We Don't Understand?

There are many conditions and disturbances of the intestinal tract we do not yet understand or cannot even classify. The IBS is not one. At present we think that it is a definite disturbance of the function of the bowel, which goes hand in hand with the symptoms described earlier. Unfortunately, many people believe that the absence of an organic cause means that the complaint is imaginary, or that the individual has brought it on him or herself, adding unnecessary guilt to suffering.

An analogy from engineering might help shed light on the different causes of physical problems. I like the way engineers use words, and the human body is surely the most complicated machine anyone has ever seen. Engineers describe disturbances in the working of an apparatus as either *structural* or *functional*. *Structural:* You step on the gas of your Rolls Royce but it does not go. Back to the factory and the fuel line is replaced: The part is defective. This is a structural defect. *Functional:* Your new stereo with all modern amplifiers is giving you static and noise instead of music from your tapes. The problem is in the fine tuning. The machine is not working properly; it needs adjusting. This is a functional problem. *Functional* does not automatically mean *psychological*. A functional disturbance of the intestine may have a psychological basis but not necessarily so; it may also be *physiological* or *biochemical* in origin. The gist of the problem is that the parts are not working properly and we need to sort out the possible reasons.

Understood in this way, the irritable bowel is a disorder in the *functioning* of the lower intestinal tract for which we have *at present no organic structural cause.* (It is possible that a basis in structure may someday be found; for years some other conditions of the colon eluded a structural account, "colonic inertia" being one.) But this is the case for IBS at present. So for the question raised at the beginning of this section, the answer is that the IBS is not a wastebasket diagnosis but a similar group of disturbances of the lower bowel, despite the individual variations that can occur in different patients.

What are IBS Patients' Most Common Complaints? How Does IBS Show Itself?

If you recognize yourself so far in this chapter, you will have some, but not necessarily all, of these disturbances:

1. Abdominal pain relieved by having a bowel movement
2. Looser and more frequent bowel movements with your abdominal pain
3. Bloated and distended abdomen, or a feeling that your abdomen is swollen
4. Some mucus in the stools
5. Very often, the most common sensation that you have not completely emptied your bowel after a movement, or what I call the "sense of incomplete evacuation"

One important sign you do not have is rectal bleeding. People with IBS can have rectal bleeding, but it's often due to trivial causes and never to IBS. It may be due to internal or external hemorrhoids (swollen, varicose veins around the rectum and anus), or a fissure (a crack or split in the lining where the rectum joins the skin around the anus) or to a more serious condition that needs looking at.

Or your symptoms may group themselves differently:

1. One group, the so-called *spastic colon* usually centers around abdominal pain in association with bowel defecation
2. Another may be *constipation* (difficulty in moving your bowels) with or without pain
3. Then there are times when you have only *painless diarrhea* ("too often and too loose" is my rough definition of diarrhea)
4. More often you swing from periods of diarrhea to those of difficulty in passing stools
5. The feeling of fullness and swelling, which in your instinctive way you feel is due to "gas": too much gas in the intestinal tract or the inability to satisfactorily pass this gas through the rectum, with or without a bowel movement.

If It's All So Simple, Why Is it so Hard to Make the Diagnosis?

Why Does My Doctor Plan so Many Tests?

The most important concern is to be sure that there is no organic basis for your symptoms and to thus rule out the possibility that you have a serious illness that mimics IBS. Difficulty in moving your bowels may be due to a mechanical blockage: a growth, small or large, benign or malignant. Diarrhea can be caused by many reasons, among them parasites and tumors that secete fluid, and pain can be caused by inflammation as well as growths.

So important is this part of the plan for your future treatment that for many doctors IBS becomes a diagnosis of exclusion: being sure that you don't have a number of conditions it would be a shame or even disastrous to overlook. Sometimes you may even think that the doctor is more concerned with conditions that you do not have than with those you do.

Furthermore, if you have a typical history of IBS, chances are that it has gone on for a long time. In this case you need to know that the underlying situation has not changed into something else or that you haven't developed a new condition that mimics the old. Finally, if you have seen blood in the bowel movements, a whole group of new conditions there must be diagnosed or disproven.

What Does the Doctor's Examination Consist Of?

The first and most important part is the story you tell your physician and the facts he or she elicits from questioning you.

Walt Whitman said that great poets need good readers. Similarly, good doctors need good patients. If you can, give your doctor your complete medical history coherently and logically in correct time sequence; if you can't, bring some notes that you have organized. For his or her part, your doctor needs to have time to listen and to ask you further questions.

Although the physical examination is important to be sure other conditions are not also present, the irritable bowel has few physical signs. You may have noticed that on the left side, in the lower quadrant of the abdomen, there may be a firm rubber hoselike structure. This is the somewhat tender sigmoid colon (the lowermost part of the large bowel before the rectum and anus, see Figure 1.2), which holds the stool before evacuation and may be the seat of chronic spasm.

What Other Tests Are Necessary?

A blood count and a search for blood in the stool (if you have not noted an obvious bleeding), easily and conveniently collected at home, are clearly in order and without any risk. Your doctor's decision to search for parasites in the stool requires a reasonable suspicion that they exist and, equally important, a laboratory your doctor trusts.

What About the More Invasive Tests?

I feel strongly that a sigmoidoscopic examination is necessary. This allows inspection of the lower portion of the bowel for 10–15 inches, with a lighted instrument introduced through the rectum, and must be preceded by proper cleansing so the observer can get a clear look (Figure 2.1). When done by an experienced person, the risk (mainly of perforation) is minimal and one that a prudent person would accept. Recent developments with flexible, fiber optic viewing devices allow a thinner, flexible instrument, known as the flexible sigmoidoscope, to be passed even further through the lower bowel (Figure 2.2). The choice here depends on your doctor's experience with these instruments.

In general, if you haven't noted bleeding, and no blood was found in a minimum of six specimens of stool, there is little need to continue tests. As with other medical conditions, however, personal health history in most individuals remains the most important basis for examination, testing, and diagnosis.

If you do have bleeding, either obvious or hidden, there is no question that you must be investigated properly to determine the source of the blood. Until recently the barium enema was the only means available. It consists of x-ray examination of the colon after filling the rectum with a barium-containing fluid, much as in an

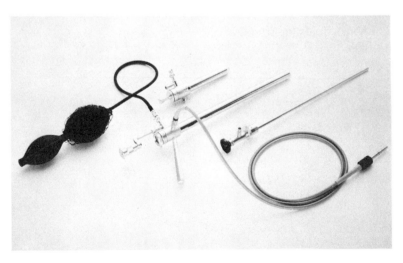

FIGURE 2.1 Rigid sigmoidoscope.

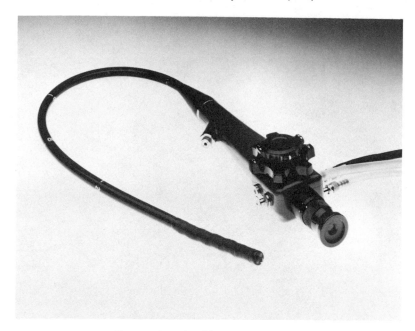

FIGURE 2.2 Flexible sigmoidoscope.

ordinary enema. Prior to this the colon must be well cleaned out by laxatives, enemas, and a special low-fiber diet. No anesthesia is needed, the discomfort is mild, and the risks extremely low. The fine detail of the pictures taken during this examination is improved if air is introduced into the rectum, so that a thin film of fluid covers the lining. This double contrast technique (air and barium fluid) (Figure 2.4) has the advantage of revealing small polyps and tiny ulcerations, but the air makes many patients quite uncomfortable. Again, the risk is minimal.

The flexible colonoscope (Figure 2.3) provides an alternate way of looking into the interior of the whole colon. Like the flexible sigmoidoscope, this instrument makes use of a flexible fiber optic system. An experienced user can insert the colonoscope from the rectum all the way around to the right side (the cecum). This, like the barium enema, requires careful cleaning out of the colon.

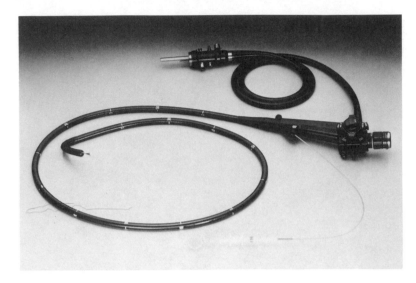

FIGURE 2.3 Flexible colonfiberscope.

Because this procedure is more uncomfortable than the barium enema, most patients are given a sedative and a pain-preventing medication by intravenous injection beforehand. This is done in an endoscopic suite either as an outpatient in a hospital, or in an endoscopist's office. There is a very small but definite risk for this procedure. Except in the presence of bleeding, I do not feel that your irritable bowel should be routinely colonoscoped, but this is a matter for individual decision by your doctor.

How Can My Irritable Bowel Syndrome Be Treated?

If we knew the cause or causes of this group of symptoms, treatment would be easier and directed at providing comfort and eliminating or avoiding the cause. This is not the case at present, however.

We do know that something has clearly disturbed the automatic functioning of the bowel, and that the search must be for possible irritants either coming from the outside or arising within the body.

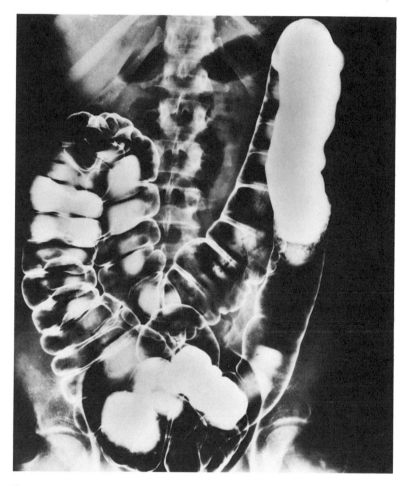

FIGURE 2.4 The colon visualized by barium enema (compare Figure 1-2).

It is natural to think first in terms of something consumed: food, drugs, antibiotics, and so on. *The refined diet* of the Western world, which is low in fiber, has been compared with the fiber-rich foods of the Third World, and the low fiber content blamed for the irritable bowel. In fact, this is far from proven nor does a high-fiber diet always improve bowel symptoms.

Food intolerance, also known as food sensitivities or food aller-gies, have always been blamed for the IBS. Many of us do have *lactose intolerance:* We cannot digest milk and milk products, especially as we grow older, because the enzyme in our intestine, lactase, which digests lactose (the sugar of milk), declines. But lactose intolerance accounts for only a few people with IBS. Recent research on food intolerances has led some investigators to suspect that wheat, dairy products, and possibly eggs cause IBS in some individuals. This approach may be helpful and is worth a trial.

Some medicines such as antibiotics and narcotics can trigger the irritable bowel, whereas some patients clearly date their problem to an attack of a "virus," causing any one of the common acute upsets of the bowel with diarrhea.

"Nerves" have always been blamed for the IBS. You may have observed a pattern in your own case of emotional upsets or stresses preceding the onset of symptoms. On the other hand, there are many beside yourself who cannot see any connection between their feelings and their gut. Yet there must be something to the general perception that brain and bowel are connected. Depression is often present and plays an important role in the whole picture. Some workers in this field have wondered whether the IBS should not be called the *irritable brain* rather than the *irritable bowel.*

More recently, doctors have looked at disturbances in the move-ments of the colon, known as motility, for different patterns. Some do indeed exist, but it is difficult to relate these disturbances (an increased or decreased amount of contraction of the colon) to the proven symptoms. Going further along this line, research has devoted much attention to detecting a disturbance in the electrical activity of the gut, with conflicting results. An electrocardiogram, which has great value in treating disturbance of rhythm of the heart, is needed for recording the electrical activity of the intestine and colon. Having taken you through this catalogue of possible factors and current ideas about IBS, you may very well ask me what my own concept is. I believe that the IBS is a disorder in the normal rhythm of the contraction and relaxation of the intestinal mus-culature apparatus, triggered off by a wide variety of irritants in your internal and external environment, for which we must hunt together.

What About the Specifics of Treatment?

Probably the most important thing a doctor can do is to reassure you about the nature of your disorder. Just knowing you do not have a serious organic disease of the colon helps a lot; although the IBS may make you uncomfortable, it will not shorten your life nor does it lead to any other disease.

What About Habits?

The Big Three

TOBACCO

There are plenty of compelling reasons for not smoking. If you smoke and suffer from IBS, you should be aware that nicotine can be an irritant. Stop smoking, using whatever technique you can find—stopping cold, "Smokenders," even hypnosis (this last one hasn't worked too often for my patients). Stopping cigarette smoking is not easy, even for highly motivated and medically informed patients, including doctors.

CAFFEINE

Since caffeine is clearly upsetting to the bowel, I think a trial of stopping all caffeine-containing beverages or food should be tried: avoid coffee, tea, chocolate, and cola drinks containing caffeine. From a food chemist I learned years ago that discarding the first cup of tea made from a fresh tea bag and drinking tea brewed from the used bag, reduces the theobromine and caffeine in the remaining cups to very low levels.

ALCOHOL

Although I am generally not opposed to moderate use of alcohol, I think a trial of stopping alcohol consumption is in order. Many patients find that wine, especially red wine, contributes to their discomfort.

Diet

Milk and Milk Products

By the time most patients get to see me with their irritable bowel symptoms, they have discovered for themselves whether they can tolerate milk and milk products. If there is any doubt, or if they have not considered this before, I suggest a 2-week trial of withdrawal of milk and milk products from their diet. Yogurt seems to be tolerated, because the organisms in yogurt supply the needed enzyme, lactase. I have not found that a lactose tolerance test, similar to a glucose tolerance test for diabetes, has helped me in this connection and so I don't subject my patients to this testing. If they are truly lactase deficient, adding the enzyme to milk may be worthwhile, since preparation of this substance (LactAid, for example) is now available.

Fiber

Hardly anyone in the Western world has not heard that fiber, bran, and other bulk-forming foods are good for the intestine. As a result everyone is eating bran muffins, adding bran to their breakfast cereals, or taking some form of plant seeds such as Metamucil to avoid constipation, diverticulosis, and cancer of the colon. As noted earlier, it is far from proven that lack of fiber is an important factor in all instances of IBS, and not everyone with IBS feels better on a high-fiber—bran diet; some may feel worse. If you are among those who have dry, hard, constipated stools, an increase in fiber is worth trying; in the diarrheal form, however, I am not convinced of its worth. The plant seeds tend to bind water and they may help in the diarrheal phases also. You may have eliminated salads and fresh fruit from your diet because you thought they might be harmful. Do not do this from theory: Convince yourself by several trials whether or not you can handle them.

Specific Foods

Many sufferers of IBS eliminate so many items from their diets because they suspect them of causing trouble that they end up eating very poor, unbalanced meals. Some patients clearly have a limited tolerance for roughage and do better when salad and some fruits are reduced or eliminated, but this can be carried too far. For example, bananas are often even well tolerated by some, especially if eaten ripe. But the haphazard elimination of one class of foods after another is to be avoided. Only repeated trials can convince you that you really cannot tolerate salad or specific fruits. Most cooked or steamed vegetables can be eaten, but some people do better if the cabbage family of vegetables is eliminated. Beans are notorious gas formers.

A few people have difficulty in handling gluten, a protein that is present in wheat, rye, oats, and barley. Gluten can cause a severe diarrheal disorder in youngsters called coeliac disease, but some adults have a limited tolerance for gluten without it being coeliac disease. In rare instances, a trial of withdrawal of these items may help.

The fear of eating specific foods because of substantial allergies of sensitivities can be carried too far and may lead to a deficient diet. In rare instances where there is a documented family history of allergies, or of allergic disorders such as hives, hay fever, or eczema, and where elimination diets do not help, I sometimes in desperation fall back on a "core" diet. For 2 or 3 weeks, I ask the patient to eat only one starch (rice); one protein (lamb or, rarely, only chicken); one fruit (canned Bartlett pears); and to drink only bottled mineral water before allowing them to add one new food at a time. Although tedious, this approach may help to pinpoint the offending food or drink.

In the age of megavitamins, it is prudent to supplement your diet with an ordinary multivitamin tablet, although high doses, which can be toxic, should be avoided. If your physician has taken you off milk and milk products, and especially if you are a woman of menopausal age, supplementary calcium will be needed.

Medicines

While drugs can't "cure" your condition, they can give you symptomatic comfort. One such group is *anticholinergics,* which block one portion of the autonomic nerves that regulate the contractions of the intestine. The basic example of this class is *atropine* or its derivates, or synthetic drugs that mimic the action of atropine. The oldest and best-known preparation of atropine is *belladonna,* taken in the form of *tincture of belladonna* in a small number of drops. Sometimes one of the anticholinergic group is combined with a general relaxer or tranquilizer (Donnatal and Librax are examples of these combinations). Capsules of *peppermint oil* are commonly used, especially in England.

Antispasmodics, which act directly by blocking nervous impulses to the intestinal muscles, also have a limited place, but give more people considerable relief (Bentyl is one such medicine).

Bulk agents (like Metamucil) may be helpful if dietary fiber and roughage do not relieve constipation. For those with disturbing amounts of diarrhea and cramps, several newer drugs, loperamide (Imodium) and diphenoxylate (Lomotil) are enjoying widespread use at present in reducing diarrhea: The first actually reduces the secretion of fluid by the intestine; the latter is related to codeine and contains atropine as well. They help by slowing down intestinal contractions.

Much research at present is focusing on the relation of the brain and the gut in an attempt to understand how one can influence the other. Chemical substances, peptides (chains of amino acids, the building blocks of protein) of identical character are present in both organs, and researchers' intuition is that they must in some way interact, so that our moods and our feelings are correlated with our bodily functions.

Some doctors feel strongly that antidepressants or mood elevating drugs help their patients (Elavil is an example of this class). Some people do not recognize that their basic mood is depression and, for them, antidepressants are very helpful.

I am not dismissing the careful, limited use of these medicines to tide you over a rough period, but they should be used sparingly to avoid your becoming dependent on them.

Handling Stress

Whatever the theories about the IBS, your experience and mine convinces us that under certain circumstances, stress—whether physical or psychological—does affect our gastrointestinal tract. This may be no different for IBS than the bad effects stress has upon any other disorder of the body: arthritis, peptic ulcer, pneumonia, tuberculosis, and so on, but it is no less real or true.

On the question of physical stress, you would agree that the proper mixture of work, play, and rest is important for good health, but no physician can write the correct prescription for you. You must solve this difficult equation yourself. But of one point I am convinced: We are born with the same neuromuscular apparatus of our ancestors who lived and evolved millions of years ago. They lived in a hostile environment where they had to fight their predators or flee them. Many of our gastrointestinal reflexes are left over from that readiness for "fight or flight." Unlike our ancestors, however, we cannot fight our "predators"—the pressures that economic responsibilities put upon us, the steps on the ladders of our careers, the unappreciative boss and the demanding public we may have to serve, the needs of aging and sick parents—nor can we flee them.

Physical exercise, however, is a good way of discharging neural and muscular tension. It is not, in my opinion, merely a matter of physical fitness but a way of releasing and getting rid of pent-up nervous energy. I am not a fanatic about this point, but you must find ways of doing some exercise. It may not be the currently-in-vogue jogging or running; walking briskly and swimming are also good forms. For tennis you may need to end up playing doubles, and for golf you may need a golf cart, but swimming you can do all your life in moderation. For the cardiovascular system (heart, lungs, and their circulation) short spurts of physical activity (20–30 minute periods three times a week) seem to be valuable. For the more continuous stress of daily living in the contemporary world, I feel that a more continuous, almost daily, program of tension-releasing exercise is better. After a stressful day, 15–20 minutes of exercise such as riding a stationary bicycle or using a rowing machine may make you fit for the evening social activities and make your gut more receptive to the evening meal.

Relaxation and Your Bowel

You may wonder why I have been stressing relaxation of the intestinal muscles so much. Patients are puzzled, worried, and even skeptical when I tell them that there is no organic basis for their abdominal pain, because it suggests that doctors have overlooked something you and they fear. "How can I have so much pain, without there being something there?"

There is something there. The pain arises from the intense contractions of the circular muscles that surround the lower bowel. If you make a fist and hold your hand contracted for 5 minutes, you will have a sore hand. Keep it contracted for 25 minutes and it will be a very sore hand. Contraction or distention of the intestines is the most powerful way of causing intestinal pain, even more than cutting the intestines. It is no wonder, then, that you have pain when your spastic bowel acts up.

How can relaxation techniques control these uncontrolled, unwished for waves of contractions, especially as these contractions are not under our will? Indeed, the actions of many of our bodily functions are under the control of our autonomic (or "automatic") nervous system, also known as the involuntary nervous system.

We have just begun to understand that certain things about our bodies, which we thought we had no control over, can be influenced and modified consciously. Blood pressure and the rate at which the heart beats seemed beyond our voluntary control. It is ironic that Westerners first called those from the East who claimed to slow down their heart rate fakirs; in their own country they called themselves fakkirs, with the entirely different meaning of healers and wise men.

Now we know that a variety of techniques can influence these apparently automatic actions of our internal organs. *TM* (transcendental meditation) has been shown to be very helpful in lowering blood pressure. Medical researchers have learned how to use the important relaxation that this method achieves without religious or semireligious ceremonies to effect the same dramatic lowering of blood pressure. Some forms of *yoga* can help the patient induce a similar form of self-relaxation. For many of us, just reading about lives and fields different from our own help achieve this inner relaxation. Cultivating one's garden, as Voltaire's Candide advised, or going fishing can induce the same desired state for some.

Paralleling these exotic techniques, current investigators are focusing on what they hope may be a more scientific approach using the technique called *biofeedback,* which you have been hearing and reading about in the semipopular press. With visual devices and simple instructions, individuals can be taught how to alter such apparently automatic responses as the temperature of the skin of the fingers by altering the flow of blood to them. Some people who have lost the control of their bowel movements have been trained to control them better by biofeedback techniques, which allow them actually to change the "tone" or state of contractions of the internal sphincter valve of the rectum, long believed beyond our conscious reach.

Biofeedback is not the first method to try to improve your IBS. If all other techniques, medicines, and dietary changes have not helped, however, it is one to consider. The course of instruction is not very long, consisting of perhaps half a dozen sessions with the biofeedback therapist to see whether you will respond. The improvement in some of my patients with this method has been quite impressive and encouraging.

Altering Your Lifestyle

In this chapter I have already emphasized that your irritable bowel is not floating freely in outer space but is attached to you and suffers the viscissitudes of your life. Although there is no one-to-one correspondence between it and your activities or feelings, in my patients, they do seem at least related. In a general way whatever is good for you will be good for your gut.

At the very least your symptoms are asking you to review your lifestyle and modify your behavior. Above I have reviewed the role of habits such as smoking, drinking, exercise, and diet. Here I want to talk about other aspects. Is your breakfast a hasty scramble because you don't allow enough time for your irritable colon to empty itself? Your timetable needs adjusting. Is your lunch a sandwich gulped down while the telephone is ringing, your associates intruding, and your secretary or the children clamoring for your attention? You will need better organization of this small oasis in your day. Must your lunch hour be spent with business colleagues from your own office? Perhaps a few moments of silence and quiet would be better in the midday. Can't you arrange to have dinner at home with your spouse after the children have had theirs? Must you lie down on the sofa right after the big evening meal? Why not sit upright in a hard-backed chair rather than on a Barcalounger or, better still, go for a walk? Need you go to sleep so soon after dinner? The stomach needs several hours to empty itself. Such ideas are simple suggestions, but they may be important for you.

Beyond these factors, your IBS is asking you if your priorities of work, play, rest, and relaxation are what you really want. I am aware of the constraints that everyday life places on each of us, but within these limits, review your priorities. You may need to trim your career goals, expected income, and social ambitions realistically. You are ambitious, but must you be vice-president in charge of everything? Are you taking on more as a suburban homemaker than you need or can handle in your child's school? I am not saying cut out from life and its stresses, but protect yourself from the unrewarding ones if you can.

A lot of books, lectures, and courses these days are directed to stress and its management. Although learning how to handle stress better and adjusting your lifestyle to your physical and psychological resources are worthwhile pursuits, my patients have not found these courses particularly helpful, because they are so general and abstract. You may need discussion and direction based on a more concrete knowledge of your particular lifestyle.

Counseling and Psychotherapy

Our discussion about altering your lifestyle in order to eliminate those irritants that are within your control leads us to the question of psychological treatment.

"Do I need a shrink? Should I contact a psychiatrist or psychotherapist because I have an irritable bowel?" These are questions I hear every day.

The experience of my patients leads me to say that a formal, orthodox psychoanalysis is not needed and, more important, really has not helped them. On the other hand, psychotherapeutic sessions with an experienced, practical, and realistic therapist, whatever the initials or letters after his or her name, may help you to discover the disturbing factors that you could manage better or avoid altogether. Talking to someone who is not your husband or wife, doctor, friend, or lover often helps to put problems in a better perspective, but be realistic about your expectations of the help you can get from psychotherapy. In an age of instant success and instant celebrities, we all want instant relief.

A more important benefit of psychotherapy may be the recognition that you are more depressed than you had realized, and that the depression is a cause or a result of your IBS. Nowadays depression is the one profound mood disturbance you ought not to suffer from, because psychotherapeutic drugs given by those who know how can drastically change the state of your feelings. Sadness, grief, loss of loved ones, must be endured and lived through, but it is the depression that does not correspond to the severity of your external problems that needs this kind of expert psychological recognition and psychotherapeutic treatment.

Probably by the time this book has been published, you will have learned that some doctors are treating the IBS with hypnosis, trying to calm down the irritable bowel by influencing the "irritable brain." There are fads and vogues in medicine as in dress, and we all want shortcuts. At the moment of writing this section, I have no personal experience with this form of treatment and need to have more published results before recommending it myself. But I do not have great confidence so far in hypnosis in modifying another form of behavior, namely smoking. So I await with some skepticism the experience of others with hypnosis in the treatment of the IBS.

Living and Living Better with the IBS: Summing It Up

In the end you can't avoid living with your irritable bowel, but neither will it shorten your life one day. Some students of the problem even believe that most persons who have the syndrome do not ever consult a doctor! If you have seen a doctor about your IBS, have been carefully but not exhaustively investigated, and found to fit this pattern of functional bowel disorders, then that knowledge will itself help you to go on enduring the symptoms, relieved of the anxiety that you have some terrible underlying disease.

In addition, once you have been alerted to the nature of your malady, you can begin to pay attention to the clues your symptoms are pointing toward. You can then try to see what patterns occur in your daily life that seem to coincide with flare-ups of the IBS. Here you will have to become Sherlock Holmes for your Dr. Watson. Review your habits: tobacco, caffeine, and alcohol—the "Big Three." Watch your eating habits carefully; some obviously need changing. Accept the fact that pills will not help too much. Do something about your failure to follow through or your good intentions to start a realistic exercise program. If you have done alone what your doctor suggests and still hurt a lot, consider getting some professional counseling or modifying your behavior, especially your destructive habits (behavioral modification therapists, these people call themselves), or even trying biofeedback techniques.

3

Inflammatory Bowel Diseases

The Serious Inflammations

Finding Out What's Wrong

You have never heard of *ileitis* or *colitis,* yet suddenly you come down with *ulcerative colitis* or your child or spouse is diagnosed as having *Crohn's disease.* Your doctor labels you or your child or spouse as having *inflammatory bowel disease* (IBD). Now wherever you go, you hear about these diseases. Other relatives or acquaintances all seem to have similar problems, yet they have different stories. Some remember that President Eisenhower had ileitis, but that he was a good general and president despite that. Everyone volunteers information. There's a foundation working on the disease. It's a viral disease. It's a psychosomatic disease. It's a Jewish disease, yet you're not Jewish and neither was President Eisenhower. What you need to know is what kind of diseases these are.

Names and Terms—General

You know at first hand that these diseases are intestinal disorders, but you need to know the meaning of the labels and words you are hearing for the first time. If you look at Figure 1.1, you will see that after you swallow a meal, it moves through the esophagus into the stomach and then into the small intestine. Although it is the longest portion of the gastrointestinal tract, the small intestine is so called because it is a narrow tube. Visualized in a gastrointestinal series after you have swallowed a mixture of water and barium, the small intestine presents the appearance of Figure 3.1. Like Gaul, the small intestine (or small bowel, as it is also known) is divided into three parts: the *duodenum,* into which the stomach empties its contents and in which the ordinary peptic ulcer occurs; the middle portion, the *jejunum* (from the Latin word for empty, since it is usually found to be empty when inspected), where foods are digested and absorbed; and the third and lowermost portion, the *ileum,* which connects the small intestine to the *colon* or *large bowel* which, though shorter than the small intestine, is much wider. Here the intestinal contents are held in storage, dried, and periodically emptied through the rectum by bowel movements. The two diseases discussed in this chapter are grouped under one umbrella term: *Inflammatory Bowel Diseases* (IBD).

Ulcerative colitis, as its name says, is an inflammation of the lining layer of any or all parts of the large bowel or colon. From Figure 1.2 you'll see that the parts of the colon are simply named: cecum (from the Latin word for blind, since this portion has a blind end), ascending, transverse, descending, and sigmoid (because of its curious curve), rectum, and anus. If the whole colon is inflamed, it is labeled *universal ulcerative colitis.* If only parts are inflamed, a specific label is used, such as *sigmoid colitis.* The word for involvement of the rectum is *proctitis.*

Crohn's disease is the other main group of IBD. It is a different kind of inflammation, which can occur anywhere in the intestinal tract from the mouth to the rectum, but is usually in the lower part of the tract. In contrast to ulcerative colitis, Crohn's disease

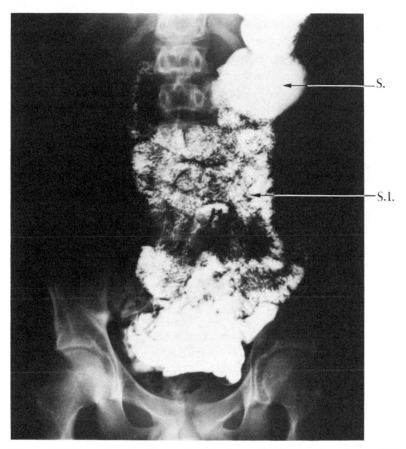

FIGURE 3.1 Gastrointestinal tract visualized by a barium meal and recorded by x-rays showing the stomach and small intestine (compare Fig 1-1). S = stomach, S.I. = small intestine.

involves the entire wall of the bowel, not only the inner lining, and has the tendency to burrow into adjacent organs. Dr. Burrill Crohn and his colleagues, Drs. Leon Ginzberg and Gordon Oppenheimer of the Mt. Sinai Hospital of New York City, first described this inflammation in the ileum in 1932, and called it *regional ileitis*. This was the form President Eisenhower had. Because we now know that this type of inflammation can occur anywhere in the intestine, and especially in the colon, we call all these varieties Crohn's disease to honor Dr. Crohn (who died recently at the extreme old age of 99!). To keep things simple we usually add the name of the part that is inflamed, so we say Crohn's ileitis or Crohn's colitis, as the case may be.

Both ulcerative colitis and Crohn's disease are *inflammatory* diseases involving parts of the bowel (bowel is used interchangeably with intestine). We all recognize an inflammation when it occurs on a part of the body we can see. For example, when skin is inflamed, it becomes reddened (because of increased flow of blood to the part), hot (again because of the blood flow), swollen (because the body mobilizes blood cells and directs them to the area to fight and contain the inflammation and carry off debris), and tender (because the nerves of the part are irritated by the local accumulation of cells and fluid). This local reaction can come to a head and form an abscess. A boil on the neck is a good example. The word *inflammation* comes from a root that means to burn, and the part of the bowel that is inflamed can be visualized as a burnt area.

Names and Terms—Specific and Nonspecific

We know the causes of a great many forms of inflammation of the bowel, but none of these has ever been linked to IBD. Parasites, such as amoeba, can cause an inflammation of the ileum and colon, which closely resembles ulcerative colitis and Crohn's disease. Bacterial infections, *Shigella, Salmonella,* and others can mimic IBD. The commonest cause of diarrhea in America at present is an infection caused by an organism carried by sick puppies, called *Campylobacter jejuni.* The colon can also become inflamed by sexually transmitted inflammations of the colon, such as gonorrhea, syphilis, herpes, and others. Your doctor should rule out all those causes before checking for IBD. We are talking about the two main groups of IBD for which we have not yet found a *specific* cause and which some doctors refer to as *nonspecific*. However, this is not a wastebasket term. The two main groups, ulcerative colitis and Crohn's disease, are separate and clearly distinct from one another.

Ulcerative Colitis

We have known about ulcerative colitis for over 100 years, longer than we have known about Crohn's disease. It is easier to diagnose and to treat, either medically or surgically, and can even be cured. Medications that can prevent recurrence are also available as long as you have a colon.

Ulcerative colitis is an inflammation of the lining of the large bowel or colon, and does not involve the small bowel except in the few cases when the inflammation washes back into the ileum. This so-called backwash ileitis has no real importance, but must be distinguished from Crohn's ileitis. Bleeding is the primary signal of ulcerative colitis, which almost always involves the rectum and may continue throughout the rest of the large bowel. Despite its name, the disease does not manifest itself as separate ulcers, but as general redness of the lining of the bowel, which bleeds easily even when gently touched. A lot of mucus and pus cover the surface, too. Ulcerative colitis is essentially a surface inflammation, although in some special circumstances it can extend through the entire thickness of the colon's wall.

Crohn's Disease

Crohn's disease, which we have known about for only a little more than 50 years, is more complicated. While it can happen in any part of the intestinal tract from the mouth to the rectum, it usually occurs in the lower bowel, the ileum, the colon, or the ileum and colon where they are joined together (see Figure 1.1). The rectum is often free of disease, but not always. Unlike ulcerative colitis, bleeding is not a hallmark of this disorder. The entire wall of the bowel becomes inflamed by the types of cells seen in chronic inflammation (lymphocytes, giant cells, eosinophiles) in contrast to the more acute types of cells in ulcerative colitis (the white blood cells of pus), and the lymph glands, which drain the intestine, become inflamed as well. Under the microscope the inflammation can be seen to consist of a special collection of cells called *granulomas;* for a while Crohn's disease was even called granulomatous colitis.

Although we can easily make the diagnosis of ulcerative colitis by looking in the rectum, we need to have x-rays of the small intestine to make the diagnosis of Crohn's ileitis. If the colon is involved, we need to look beyond the rectum with the newer flexible fiber optic viewing systems, which enable us to thread our way from the rectum around the colon to the cecum (see Figure 2.3). Crohn's disease has one other characteristic feature. The inflammation is deeper than the surface layer, and can track through the wall of the bowel and burrow into neighboring organs and even reach through to the skin. These burrowing tracts are called *fistulas* and are frequently found about the rectum.

The General Nature of IBD

What do we know about these two diseases that might help us understand their nature? Although they are found throughout the world, they are concentrated in the developed countries; they are diseases of affluence and relatively new ones. They appear to be diseases of the city, not the country.

Men and women share them equally. All races and classes are involved; blacks are now no longer exempt. In some families, more than one member may have one or more forms of IBD, and close blood relatives have more than their share of similar illnesses than would be expected by chance. You don't have to be Jewish, as I have said, yet in the United States and Western Europe, a preponderance of Jews have ulcerative colitis and Crohn's disease. In the

United States and western Europe, this may be as much as three times more than the non-Jewish population.

Sufferers do not have more of the so-called psychosomatic diseases, such as peptic ulcer, than might be expected. Although the annual number of new cases of ulcerative colitis has remained unchanged since we began keeping good statistics, in Crohn's disease the number has been increasing, although it may have leveled off lately. For a while it seemed that Crohn's disease had assumed almost epidemic proportions.

Although Crohn's disease and ulcerative colitis can be diagnosed at any age, they typically attack the adolescent and young adult, but a second peak of attacks does occur in a smaller number of persons later in life, centering around the age 50. They can appear mysteriously in people who have been very healthy before. They may creep up on the patient or may suddenly explode. The symptoms may be more or less continuous or subside for long periods, so that the patient returns to his or her previous state of health. Episodes may be triggered by an infection, antibiotics, stress (whether it is physical or psychological), or may have no clear-cut cause. The important point to remember is that both diseases respond to medications that suppress inflammation. Although removing the diseased tissue in ulcerative colitis can permanently cure it, this is not the case in Crohn's disease. Removing the diseased tissue in Crohn's disease, however, usually dramatically improves the patient's health and quality of life.

Can we predict who will come down with these diseases, especially since more than one family member may have them? We have no way of telling in advance who is susceptible, because the defects in these patients' immune system (which are present in some but by no means in all) may be, I suspect, the result rather than the cause of the disease, and there are no known genetic markers. Of all the thousands and even millions of patients with these diseases, less than a handful of husbands or wives have developed it from their spouses after living together for years; IBD is not easily communicable. So far, laboratory research has not found the cause of either IBD, and no confirmed success has followed attempts to give these diseases to animals, although some animals have diseases that resemble ileitis and colitis. The cotton top marmoset has a disease in captivity that closely resembles ulcerative colitis, even to the extent of developing cancer of the colon after a chronic course. A tremendous amount of effort is presently being devoted to finding the cause(s) of IBD. My guess (and it is only a guess) is that these disorders, especially Crohn's, behave like infectious diseases. They may resemble the so-called slow viruses, which require years to work their effects, have never been seen under the microscope or grown in the test tube, but can be transmitted to the right animal species. I would also guess that the agents of IBD need a susceptible population, which may be genetically determined, and exert their effects by disturbing the susceptible individual's immune system.

How Do These Diseases Show Themselves?

So far I have talked about ulcerative colitis and Crohn's disease together. Now when I discuss the way these disorders affect the patient, I will have to separate them because they behave differently in many respects.

Ulcerative Colitis

Ulcerative colitis starts by inflaming the lining in the lowest portion of the rectum. Rectal bleeding is the most striking, frequent, and important sign. The bleeding may range from mild to severe, and the color of the blood may vary from bright red to darker shades. The blood may show on the toilet paper, in the bowl, or on the stool. Because the bleeding is often painless, the individual may wonder if he or she has hemorrhoids or piles. The bleeding need not be associated with marked changes in bowel habits, which may in fact be perfectly normal. Frequently, though, the individual notices a slight change in bowel habits, usually a slight increase in the number or in the wateriness of the bowel movement; if the latter, it is not watery enough to be considered diarrhea. However, several loose diarrheal stools may also be the way the disease shows up.

These signs describe *proctitis,* the mildest form of ulcerative colitis and the one that occurs in the rectum.

Individuals with proctitis are not very sick. They feel well and can carry on their usual activities. In other individuals in whom the disease is either slow or sudden in coming on, the signs and symptoms are much more dramatic. They feel sick, have more diarrhea, lose their appetite, lose weight, and run a fever that may be only low grade. They also have pain that appears as a cramping sensation in the lower left side of the abdomen. When these general sensations are present, we can be sure we are dealing with more than the local mild inflammation in the rectum of proctitis. Now we are dealing with an inflammation that has extended to a good part of the left side of the colon. Since individuals with proctitis are not very sick, they tolerate the condition for a long time. Only the persistence and recurrence of bleeding leads them to seek medical help. The sicker individuals with left-sided colitis do not put up with their complaints for very long and consult doctors earlier.

People with universal ulcerative colitis are quite sick. They run fever, lose their appetite, stop eating, and lose weight. They have lots of diarrhea, which keeps them up at night, and a great deal of pain, which is diffused all over the abdomen. They bleed a lot, sometimes in clots, and not necessarily in association with bowel movements. These are the dramatic and fortunately rarer forms of ulcerative colitis. In many people, universal ulcerative colitis develops insidiously. On rare occasions these individuals may develop a marked swelling of the abdomen and of the intestines and a sudden paralysis of all activity of the colon. This is called "toxic dilation of the colon." These individuals need prompt emergency care to ward off perforation of the colon.

Crohn's Disease

Although the symptoms of the different kinds of ulcerative colitis resemble each other and vary only in severity, the presentation of Crohn's disease is more complicated. The typical form is seen in a young person who develops pain in the right side of the abdomen, a low-grade fever, and perhaps experiences some minor changes in bowel movements. He or she is suspected of having appendicitis and is operated on only to be discovered to have a normal appendix. They do have an area of thickened, inflamed bowel, however, which the surgeon recognizes, even without a biopsy, as Crohn's disease. The area involved is usually the ileum. Occasionally it may be the ileum and the tip of the cecum.

Another textbook picture is the young person, between the ages of 16 and 20, with a history of bellyaches, periods of diarrhea alternating with periods of constipation, who has for several years been thought to have a "nervous stomach" or an irritable colon. Then some complications develop, such as fever, tenderness in the abdomen, perhaps now, for the first time, bleeding, and a swelling in the right lower abdomen, which the doctor calls a mass. These complications often take place when the patient goes off to college for the first time, perhaps in a setting of stress. Now the possibility arises that he may have Crohn's disease, which x-rays then confirm.

The third often-seen situation is when a young adolescent fails to grow, mature sexually, or has a delay in the onset of menstruation. In some of these cases the question of Crohn's disease does not even arise because intestinal symptoms are not in the forefront of the clinical picture, and the mild diarrhea and pain may not even bother the patient. However, astute pediatricians and internists recognize that Crohn's disease can delay maturation.

Another characteristic situation arises when a youngster, anywhere from ages 10 to 20, without many previous intestinal symptoms, develops an abscess or fistula around the rectum. Because this person has no real history of intestinal difficulty, little intestinal investigation has been done, especially since rectal pain often prevents this and the abscess is simply incised and drained by a surgeon. When the wound fails to heal and continues to drain, then the physician suspects for the first time that the fistula is a signal of more serious trouble upstream. The appropriate tests are now done, which reveal Crohn's disease either in the small or large bowel. These abscesses or fistulae can present themselves for the first time in the Bartholin glands, which surround the vagina. Rectal bleeding, whose severity at times can be quite alarming to the patient and physician, can occur in Crohn's disease, although rarely is it the only sign. It may take more extensive tests to prove that bleeding is the result of Crohn's disease higher up in the intestine.

A characteristic complaint of people with Crohn's disease is the obstruction of the intestine, which develops slowly after many years of diarrhea. Ironically, this results from the narrowing and scarring of the intestines, which has taken place during healing. President Eisenhower was operated on not because of his ileitis, but because the passageway of his intestine had become extremely narrowed. Individuals with an obstructed intestine do not feel sick in general; they have a good appetite and run no fever because the inflammation is not active. It is the scarring that causes the difficulty. Such "mechanical" problems have the best therapeutic results, since they are easily corrected by surgically removing the scar.

IBD Can Cause Trouble Outside the Intestines: Extraintestinal Manifestations

Inflammatory bowel diseases affect the intestine, yet they can also cause problems outside the intestinal tract. These curious problems are disturbing to the patient and very frequently not connected by either doctor or patient to the underlying disease, yet they are related and almost all are treatable. These extraintestinal manifestations occur in both ulcerative colitis and Crohn's disease. They are important in themselves because of the distress they cause and also because they can call attention to either intestinal disease, which may have been overlooked yet requires attention. Treating the intestinal disease heals the extraintestinal manifestations. The difficulty is that they are extensive, and appear when the intestinal inflammation is active and subside when it quiets down. They may reach from the head to the toe.

The individual with Crohn's disease or ulcerative colitis may develop conjunctivitis, which usually occurs in only one eye.

Inflammation of the iris may also occur. Crops of canker sores in the mouth may herald an attack of Crohn's disease.

Other people with an IBD may have a variety of skin conditions. One of them is erythema nodosum (literally, red bumps) which appears on both shins. Various rashes can suddenly develop anywhere on the skin as well as very ugly infected sores, which are called pyoderma gangrenosum, especially on the lower legs. These respond to whatever makes the colon and ileum better.

Joint pains may often be the first and for years the only extraintestinal problem a sufferer of IBD experiences. Aches of the wrists, fingers, knees, and ankles, which sometimes develop into red, swollen, hot joints are easier to treat than pains located in the spine or pelvic bones. This is not a chronic deforming type of arthritis, like rheumatoid arthritis, and individuals need not fear crippling. Some people with Crohn's disease may develop stiffness in the spine and low back pain. Sometimes the skin disease psoriasis and the arthritis of Crohn's disease go together, but we don't know why.

Today we think the extraintestinal manifestations of ulcerative colitis and Crohn's disease arise because the inflamed intestine releases certain protein substances called antigens, against which the body forms antibodies, and that these antigen-antibody couples float around in the blood and settle in the eye, the skin, or the joints and cause the difficulties.

Patients and families ought to know that on some occasions extraintestinal manifestations may occur in patients with marked disturbances in the small intestine, particularly the ileum, either because it is the seat of disease or because of surgery in that area. These curious complications, which are difficult to relate to the underlying disease at first glance, include gallstones and kidney stones. They need care in their own right and may occasionally call attention to the fact that the patient does have Crohn's disease.

When to Go to the Doctor, and What Kind

From time to time we all get some lower abdominal distress: belly-aches, cramps, gripping in the tummy, or loosening of our bowels;

we feel sick and may have a low-grade fever. We pass it off as "something I ate," "an intestinal virus," or it goes away by itself, and we feel well enough to resume our usual activities and diet.

Inflammatory bowel diseases are different: they linger, or if they subside by themselves, they return again. We begin to realize that we can't be having so many "viruses" so frequently, and if we generally feel sick, lose our appetite and weight, and experience persistent abdominal pain, we know something definite is wrong which needs looking after.

There is one symptom that we cannot and dare not pass off, hoping it will go away by itself, however. This is rectal bleeding. Of course bleeding with bowel movements can have a trivial cause: a hemorrhoid, dilated veins at the end of the rectum (known as a pile), a fissure (a painful crack at the end of the rectum), an acute bacterial infection of the colon or, more rarely, a true intestinal virus. By now doctors have made everyone aware that rectal bleeding is also a warning of a cancer in the rectum. The lower down the affected part of the intestine, the redder and brighter the color of the blood. If you experience rectal bleeding, or return or persistence of the symptoms outlined above, you ought to consult a doctor, preferably your own doctor who knows you, your family, and your medical history. These days, however, many of us do not have a family doctor. If you don't, find a good general practitioner or an internist. Do not assume offhand your problem is a rectal one and think that you need a proctologist—a specialist with a surgical leaning who deals with diseases of the rectum and anus.

Because of your family's medical history, or what you have read, or fears that you may have the serious kind of inflammation of the bowel described in this chapter, you may think you ought to consult a specialist in intestinal illnesses—a gastroenterologist. You may want to and, perhaps, even need to, but let your general doctor see you first, decide whether he or she will make the diagnosis, do the necessary examination, and plan the treatment before you see one or more specialists. Your general health picture needs to be taken into account first.

What Is the Heart of the Doctor's Examination?

In addition to a general physical, what tests and examinations should you expect to undergo to establish the diagnosis of some form of inflammatory bowel disease?

A rectal examination by the finger is needed first to rule out a cancer of the rectum. A look at the lining of the lower part of the rectum is the next step. In this examination, known as a proctoscopy, the physician inserts a small-diameter instrument into the rectum, which allows him or her to look at the degree of inflammation of the lining membrane, the mucosa, and need not be preceded by a cleansing enema, although some physicians prefer that the patient have a tap water enema, or a Fleets enema beforehand. Only slightly uncomfortable, this form of looking into the interior of the intestinal tract is a very safe procedure.

If there is no observable bleeding at the time of the examination, your doctor should check your stool for hidden chemical bleeding. In addition, the stool should be tested for abnormal bacteria and for eggs of the adult forms of intestinal parasites. Finally, your doctor will want a blood count to detect anemia and a sedimentation rate test to measure the degree of inflammation.

The physician has the option of inspecting the lower bowel further by using a rigid sigmoidoscope, or the more flexible endoscope. The latter contains a fiber optic system, which allows light to be bent easily as the instrument goes further into the alimentary canal. Here the doctor's experience with the instrument at his or her disposal is important. As with a proctoscopy, cleansing enemas are in order to clear the way for an undisturbed view of the mucosa.

Usually the diagnosis of some variant of ulcerative colitis can be made simply by inspecting the inflamed mucosa, and verified by the absence of all the organisms and bacteria that can mimic this disorder. Examination of the whole colon endoscopically (a colonoscopy) is not necessary at this point, nor is examination of the colon by barium enema. If the proctoscope and/or the sigmoidoscope (flexible or rigid) reveal a normal lower bowel, however, then barium studies are needed to search for evidence of Crohn's disease. These studies consist of a gastrointestinal series and small bowel series with films that follow through the remainder of the colon.

What Are the Risks of These Essential Examinations?

The rectal examination, proctoscopy, stool cultures, and smears for chronic bleeding present no real risks to the patient.

Sigmoidoscopy with rigid or flexible scopes carries a small but acceptable risk of perforation in ulcerative colitis. In mild cases in which a proctoscopy reveals obvious inflammation, sigmoidoscopy does not seem warranted. In severely ill patients, the risk of perforation is too great and is not acceptable. In these instances, colonoscopy is entirely out of order, and the same holds true for examination of the colon by barium enema. An examination of the stomach, small bowel, and even colon with barium given by mouth has virtually no risk, but it may be difficult for the individual to pass all the barium contrast mixture with the stool if there is any scarred narrowing of the gut.

At times it may be necessary to perform a biopsy of the lining mucosa of the rectum or of the adjacent area, the sigmoid colon, in order to aid in the diagnosis. Biopsy usually presents little risk of perforation, but bleeding may occur at the biopsy site and be somewhat difficult to stop. Doctors who do biopsies must be prepared to control the bleeding, and the patient should have proper blood studies beforehand to guard against unknown defects in the blood clotting system.

How Sure Can We Be About the Diagnostic Label?

If your doctor has done the basic tests and examination outlined above, you can be reasonably confident about the correctness of the diagnosis—no trivial point considering the possible seriousness of your disease. Labels can be wrong, however, if the search for odd bacteria and parasites is not thorough or a history of antibiotic treatment for other infections just prior to the IBD is overlooked.

Very important is the fact that at the beginning of an attack, the colitis may actually be what its name indicates: "an acute self-limited colitis." As a result, your doctor cannot always predict whether the colitis will go away by itself, never to return, or be chronic.

Rarely, the diagnosis of IBD will be missed because the sigmoidoscopy and even the x-rays of your colon are not helpful. If IBD is strongly suspected and your stool contains red or white blood cells, your doctor may perform a colonoscopy to find a "segmental" colitis—a patch of inflammation not seen on the x-ray or sigmoidoscopy.

Your doctor may suspect that you have Crohn's disease of the small bowel if your symptoms are typical, but the x-ray and test may not reveal any disease. Although there probably are times when the disease is present but not visible on x-ray, I feel it is a mistake to tell a person that he or she has Crohn's disease without x-ray evidence, because it is such a serious diagnosis.

Once the Diagnosis of IBD Is Made

You have just been told by your doctor that you have one of the inflammatory bowel diseases (IBD). In most cases your doctor can tell you which of the two main kinds of IBD you have: ulcerative colitis or Crohn's disease. Occasionally, the diagnosis is uncertain until the course of the disease makes clear which of the two it is. This uncertainty should not make you anxious, because these disorders closely resemble each other and the ways of treating them are often similar.

Along with the relief of knowing that the cause of your pain, diarrhea, rectal bleeding, and weakness is not due to a malignant tumor, comes dismay on hearing that the causes of these diseases are still unknown. The patient and those concerned about him or her need to know that on the whole these two illnesses need not shorten the patient's life by one day. Further, they may disappear as mysteriously as they appeared. Finally, the body affected by IBD has a real capacity to heal itself, and doctors try to mobilize this defense machinery.

How can the body overcome a disorder whose cause is unknown and for which there is no specific cure? It does so by the same mechanisms it uses to fight diseases whose causes are known and for which a remedy exists. Even in pneumococcal pneumonia treated with penicillin, it is the body's own defense mechanisms, the white blood corpuscles, which gobble up the bacteria. In the inflammatory bowel diseases, it is the body's own resistance, mobilized in its cells and antibodies factors, which protects against the invasion of the inflammation. Everything the doctor does to treat the patient is directed toward strengthening the body's resistance against the inflammation and to tilt the balance in the patient's favor. Although each is important by itself, it is the combined effect of diet, medicines, lifestyle modification, and psychological treatment that can make the difference in treating these diseases.

Treating These Diseases Means Total Management of Life with IBD

An important point to make is that a person's inflamed intestinal tract is not floating free in outer space; it is attached to and part of that person. Although some doctors believe they are treating a case of disease, others believe they are treating a specific person with an illness. The latter approach can be summed up thus: Anything that is good for the patient will be good for the gut!

Habits: The Big Three

What role do they play in helping or retarding recovery or improvement?

CIGARETTE SMOKING

Patients often blame their colitis or ileitis on giving up cigarette smoking. I have heard this several times and so have other physicians who treat many patients with IBD. I'm not yet convinced that this is more than a coincidence and certainly do *not* recommend resuming smoking or starting smoking in anyone, least of all in young patients whose illness may last for some time. I don't have to preach the case against smoking in general; it's clear-cut and unarguable. Not only can smoking depress the capricious appetite of people who have IBD, but in all patients, nicotine, I believe, can have a bad effect on the blood flow in the intestines.

CAFFEINE

In many people a cup of coffee, which contains 40–50 milligrams of caffeine, stimulates a bowel movement. (Although tea contains less caffeine, it does have other substances of the same chemical family.) It doesn't make sense to take caffeine-containing beverages, including the cola family of drinks, if you're already having too many bowel movements, but I am not fanatical about this point in general.

ALCOHOL

Alcohol plays a large role in the social and business life of Western countries. It is probably the most widely used tranquilizer. Moderate alcohol intake is believed to help the circulation, especially the coronary arteries of the heart, and to increase certain positive factors against heart disease in the blood (high-density lipoproteins, "HDL," which we all read about in the daily newspapers and magazines). Alcohol does have deleterious effects on the subtle digestive enzymes of the intestinal lining. When my patients are sick, I favor reduction or elimination of alcohol, although I would not forbid some alcohol in the form of wine to stimulate the capricious appetite of an adult accustomed to drinking. When a patient with Crohn's disease is being treated with the drug called metronidazole (Flagyl), alcohol is completely out. A severe reaction may occur, which resembles the effect of an alcoholic drink on someone who is being treated with Antabuse for alcoholism. These reactions can be serious and alarming.

Diet

Diet probably causes more discontent and confusion in the minds of the patient and the family than about any other part of today's medical treatment of IBD. We all have the instinctive feeling that food must play some part in helping or hindering the health of our intestines, yet doctors, including specialists in this field, often seem vague or lackadaisical in their dietary instructions.

We know that certain intestinal diseases are caused or influenced by too much or too little of a particular food or type of food. Coeliac disease in children is an excellent example. Eliminating one specific protein, gluten, from the diet stops this diarrheal disease. Doctors forbid wheat, rye, oats, and barley, as in the old nursery rhyme, and insist that their patients' families read the labels on prepared foods. Unfortunately, it is not so simple in IBD. No one knows of any specific food or foods the patients lack or take too much of. So doctors sound too permissive or unconcerned when they tell IBD patients to eat "whatever agrees with you."

Yet nutrition does play an important part in getting better. The clearest case is the child with Crohn's disease or ulcerative colitis who is not growing because of the disease or the medication. Increasing the number of calories the child takes in will lead to marked improvement not only in weight, but in growth and sexual development.

If you consider the fact that the inflamed lining of the sick intestine does not absorb food as efficiently as it should, and that this same delicate membrane leaks fluid like a burned skin and allows some blood to leak out, then you will realize that diet can and does play a part in taking care of these diseases. Because the patient with these disorders often has a poor appetite and because there is so much folklore about food, it is no wonder that patients end up with lopsided and faddish diets.

The necessity of a well-balanced, nutritious diet is all the more important for these sick people who must try to get the basic elements of a good diet into them. They need a high protein intake to

make up for any lack of proteins as well as for healing their intestinal wound: egg, cheese, cereals, chicken, fish, and meat, together
with vegetables. Remember that a high-protein diet is a weight
reduction diet, so that the protein calories must be balanced by an
increased amount of starches: potatoes, rice, spaghetti, noodles,
bread, and cakes. Fat should not be automatically eliminated. Fat
gives the body 9 calories for each gram of food eaten, whereas
protein and starch give only 4. Vitamins are needed, especially
because the intake of vitamin C is reduced since raw fruits (especially citrus fruits and salads) are frequently cut back if not cut out of
the patient's diet.

The questions I am most often asked have to do with dairy
products, roughage (raw fruits, salad, and cooked vegetables), and
vitamin supplements. The most important point to remember is
that your past food experience, your tolerance and intolerance of
certain foods, must be taken into account. If your past history has
shown a clear-cut intolerance for a specific food, or a class of foods,
discuss this with your doctor. You are not supposed to leave outside his or her consultation room what you have learned about
yourself in the past, but be sure that you are convinced not by one
bad experience but by careful observations over a long time.

LACTOSE AND DAIRY PRODUCTS

Patients and doctors for a long time have thought and wondered
whether dairy products are bad for patients with IBD. Some have
even suggested that patients weaned too early from breast milk or
not breast-fed may have a greater tendency to have colitis, but this
notion has not stood up. However, intolerance to lactose, the sugar
of milk, rather widespread in the general population, increases as
we become older, because the intestinal enzyme lactase, which
splits the two parts of lactose, diminishes with age. This leads to the
undigested and unabsorbed lactose (milk sugar) getting into the
lower intestine, with the bacteria going to work on this material.
Cramps, bloating, gas, and passage of loose, watery, and at times
foul stools follow. Any extensive inflammation in the small intestine, where this enzyme is located, will almost certainly lead to not

enough lactase to do the normal job. Small areas of inflammation are not important in this regard.

Some people are intolerant to other elements in milk, the proteins (casein and lactalbumin). By the time I get to see patients with ulcerative ileitis and colitis, most have already discovered whether dairy products make a difference: whether they increase the discomfort and lead to diarrhea and cramps and, in some cases, even to increased blood in the stools. If their experience convinces me and them that they cannot tolerate these products, I advise stopping them. If there is any uncertainty or past history of milk intolerance in childhood, I suggest a short course of a low-lactose diet to decide this point.

I have not found that testing the patient with a lactose tolerance test helps me. In this test, which is like a glucose tolerance test (the sugar tolerance test for diabetes), bloods are taken after the patient has a large dose of lactose by mouth. Rather, the ability of the patient to tolerate dairy products in the course of real life is much more useful. If there really is lactose intolerance, this means that the patient should avoid milk, cheese, ice cream, and butter only. I am not convinced that lactose incorporated into prepared foods is important, and I don't advise parents to read the labels on food for the lactose content. For those on such a low-lactose diet, there is no substitute for cheese and most ice creams, although some lactose-free ice creams are beginning to appear commercially. Some margarines contain milk solids, so here one must read the labels. For milk, nondairy creamers can be substituted. If this ritual does not have a clear-cut effect in 2 weeks, I abandon it and suggest a relatively slow return of their intake.

If, after this dietary trial, you and the doctor have a feeling that it is useful, you might consider the use of the commercially available lactase-treated milk (LactAid, for example) to see whether this treated milk is tolerated and worth the effort. Also, intolerance for dairy products may not be all or none: You might be able to tolerate a small amount, but not a very large amount. These are some of the things to do to help decide whether it is worthwhile remaining on a low-lactose diet for an indefinite period of time.

ROUGHAGE AND FIBER

Everyone nowadays knows that one ought to have a good intake of fresh fruits and vegetables as well as cereal grains, because our Western diet is too refined. Everyone has read over and over again in the popular press that in certain parts of the world (Africa), where people eat loads of roots and fibers, the population does not suffer from any of the intestinal disorders we have in America: spastic colon, irritable colon, constipation, diverticulitis, and even cancer of the colon. This is true, but it would be simple-minded to believe that this is due only to the high fiber in those native populations. They don't have any environmental pollution, as well as the IRS and food additives, among other things. Be that as it may, a diet adequate in fiber is a healthy one.

However healthy this kind of diet may be in general, when you are sick with diarrhea and have abdominal cramps with active bleeding, it makes no sense to push to eat large amounts of raw fruits and vegetables. At these times, the diet should contain cooked vegetables and canned fruits. Bananas are usually tolerated when they are ripe. Among the steamed and cooked vegetables, I would skip the cabbage family (cabbage, brussels sprouts, broccoli, and cauliflower), although florets of broccoli seem to be well tolerated. Potatoes and whole-wheat (whole meal) bread supply some fiber as well. On the other hand, if you can tolerate them, and only trial and error can tell, then you ought to be allowed to attempt to eat some limited amounts of fresh fruits and salads, unless there is an area in the intestine that is narrowed by previous inflammation and a tight scar. In these instances it would be foolhardy to run the risk of blocking such a narrowed area and being completely obstructed. I have seen such scarred areas become blocked by corn-on-the-cob, a swallowed peach pit, and even by a number of pimento stuffed jumbo olives!

VITAMINS, FOOD SUPPLEMENTS, MINERALS, AND TRACE ELEMENTS

Patients, their families, and doctors are overwhelmed by a flood of press regarding the role of accessory food factors, the vitamins, in treating IBD. What do we know that makes sense and what pills is it reasonable to take? For the patient eating a complete, normal, well-balanced diet, the problems that arise depend on whether he is digesting and absorbing the elements of his food properly. Since there is always some doubt about this in the patient with ileitis and colitis, it is reasonable to supplement the presumably normal intake with a multivitamin of any standard brand. Because fresh fruits and vegetables as well as fruit juices are the first to be eliminated from the patient's diet, supplementation with vitamin C (ascorbic acid) is in order. Since dairy products are almost always routinely reduced or eliminated, a lack of calcium may result. To make up for this, be sure that the calcium is not taken in the form of lactose (calcium lactate), which would defeat the purpose of reducing lactose in the diet.

Patients become anemic (that is, have a low hemoglobin and red blood cell count) from several causes: rectal bleeding, inadequate intake of iron, and the blood forming folic acid and vitamin B_{12}, failure to absorb vitamin B_{12} in the ileum, failure to absorb iron in the duodenum, and because one of the drugs widely used in treating IBD, sulfasalazine, interferes with absorption of folic acid. Your doctor can check the blood levels of vitamin B_{12} and folate, as well as the levels of iron in the blood. Based on these tests, vitamin B_{12} can be given by injection to avoid the problem of absorption; folic acid can be given in pill form by mouth, and iron can be replaced either by pills to be swallowed or, if need be, by some preparation for injection.

In my experience, many patients with IBD have some abdominal distress if they take iron by mouth, especially cramps and constipation. The black color it gives the stool may be confused with blood. It may be necessary to try a few preparations of iron before finding one that does not give you any trouble.

There are some vital substances that circulate in the blood in very small amounts, so-called "trace elements," which are important for the body's tissues to function properly. The best known generally at present is zinc; some patients have skin and mouth problems as well as intestinal problems because their stores of zinc are low. These are patients who have been nutritionally depleted by starvation, inadequate intake of food, or because of intake of intravenous fluids lacking the proper amount of zinc. For these patients zinc can be given in a pill form. A rare form of depletion is the lack of the element selenium, which causes heart trouble, because patients have been given all their nutrition by vein (so-called total parenteral hyperalimentation). This is now being corrected by including selenium in the solutions used to feed these sick patients.

Because the patients may have capricious appetites, or because longstanding habits of poor eating interfere with their needed nutrition, food supplements are available to try to get them to take in sufficient calories and nutrients. Some fluid preparations high in calories and pleasantly flavored can be offered to the patients to supplement their limited intake, but not in place of real food, unless there is such mechanical blockage in the gut that regular food cannot get by.

Diet in General

The important moral of this entire discussion on diet and IBD is that every effort should be made to have the patient take an attractive-looking, palatable, general diet, bearing in mind that IBD is not caused or cured by a specific diet. Mealtime should be a pleasant experience, not a medical hassle. In some special instances when resting the bowel may be helpful, it is now possible to give patients all their nutritional requirements, including calories, by vein. This can be carried out at home, and often at night if the patient is up and about by day, and can be supplied by nutritional support services and companies. Although this is not a permanent cure, this form of nutritional support (TPN, as Total Parenteral Nutrition is abbreviated) is an important modern and recent advance in living with ileitis and colitis.

Medications

Most of the medications used in treating IBD patients are the same for both Crohn's disease and ulcerative colitis, so I shall discuss them here together. They fall into two main groups: those that are intended to reduce the inflammation of the bowel, the "antiinflammatory group," and those that we use to make the patient more comfortable, the "symptomatic" group of drugs.

Antiinflammatory Medicine

SULFASALAZINE

Probably the most widely used drug of this group is sulfasalazine (salazopyrine), best known under the trade name of Azulfadine. It is a combination of an aspirin-related compound, 5 aminosalicylic acid (5 ASA) and a sulfa compound, sulfapyridine. This medication, taken by mouth, is split in two by the bacteria in the bowel, and we think the 5 ASA is the part that does the patient good. Most of sulfasalazine or its split products remain in the intestine and are excreted in the stools. One need not worry about the kidney with this drug, and while patients often think they need to drink loads of water, this is not the case. Like all drugs, sulfasalazine may have side effects. Generally, they are really quite trivial, although the patient may be very uncomfortable. They are mainly headache, nausea, and loss of appetite.

I use these drugs by starting with small doses instead of a large amount, and building up slowly, hoping in this way to avoid the nausea and loss of appetite. Most patients adapt to and develop a tolerance for sulfasalazine. Some do not. With these relatively few, the coated form may help, and often a simple antihistamine may smooth over the unpleasant side effects. More serious side effects include fever, rash, and jaundice. There seems to be no simple test at present for predicting who will have these side effects, which may appear at any time in the course of the use of the drug. I have mentioned that a patient taking Azulfadine needs more folic acid than usual, and a possible side effect of the drug requires that blood counts be done at regular intervals. Newer preparations of the active principle (5 ASA) are now being developed and tried in patients to avoid side effects and may be commercially available by the time you read this.

Azulfadine is a very useful drug in treating ulcerative colitis and Crohn's disease. In addition, in ulcerative colitis it can help to prevent recurrences and minimize the chances of their reoccurring. You can shorten the duration of recurrences by keeping on the drug even when feeling well and in remission, since ulcerative colitis tends to recur. Unlike steroids (cortisone derivatives), which will be discussed next, sulfasalazine has the advantage of being able to be stopped abruptly without any withdrawal symptoms, should that be necessary.

STEROIDS

Steroids are synthetic medications that resemble the secretions of the cortex (the outer rim) of the adrenal glands. They are powerful drugs that suppress inflammation. Accordingly, they are widely used in both ulcerative colitis and Crohn's disease. They take hold rapidly, suppress fever, stimulate appetite, and reduce the inflammation of the bowel. They clearly make the patient feel better, and are extremely useful medicines. They can be given by mouth, as well as injected under the skin or into veins. They can also be placed in the rectum in suppositories or instilled into the rectum and lower bowel in a liquid form via an enema or in an aerosol. In addition, the patient's own adrenal cortex can be stimulated to secrete its own adrenal hormones by using the drug ACTH, derived from the front part of the pituitary gland, the master gland of the brain, which then secretes the adrenocorticotropic hormone (ACTH). These have the same benefits as the steroids themselves but without symptoms of withdrawal, because ACTH has not made the adrenal glands hibernate. These also have the same side effects.

On the other hand, these steroids have their own limitations. Because they suppress the normal secretions of the adrenal cortex needed to sustain life in every cell in the body, they cannot be stopped abruptly. If they are, a serious condition of adrenal suppression and insufficiency results. In some patients, slow withdrawal leads to withdrawal symptoms similar to those of narcotic withdrawal. Tapered slowly, steroids can be safely lowered without serious problems.

In medicine as elsewhere, however, one gets nothing for nothing. The good effects of steroids are not outweighed by their undesirable side effects. Most, fortunately, are reversible when the drug is stopped. Some are purely cosmetic: retention of fluid; swelling of the face, hands, and ankles (managed by watching one's salt intake and not eating salty foods); and the growth of downy hair on the faces of female patients. This hair should not be plucked or removed by electrolysis, but simply bleached by peroxide, because it will disappear by itself after the patient comes off the drug. In some individuals, fat is laid down between the shoulder blades.

The more serious side effects occur when the patient is on a high dose of cortisone drugs for a long period of time. It is the patient who has been treated for a long time who develops a cataract or an ulcer of the stomach or softening of the bones. If taken late in the evening, cortisone keeps some awake. Most patients feel better on steroids, and a few develop a "high"; in them it brings out the underlying personality with its attendant anxieties. Despite these side effects and the fact that some steroids can cover up acute abdominal symptoms, this class of medicine is useful and widely used. My only advice to all patients is to have them remind their doctors of any peculiar symptoms they may be having, and to try to get off the drug as soon as possible, even if reducing the drug does not suppress all the symptoms. It is better to tolerate a few symptoms without steroids than to suppress them all and require long-term usage of large doses of steroids. Here your own contribution to your well-being involves not insisting on remaining on a drug that makes you feel so much better, but that carries with it real hazards if used for too long.

Some attention must be paid to the fact that steroids can retard growth in children. Again this must be balanced against the beneficial effect of the drugs on the child's illness, in the hope that the beneficial effects will outweigh the deleterious ones. In the long run these children do have a spurt of growth and catch up. So, while I do not push parents to allow me to use steroids in children, one is often driven to that extreme because of the need for short-term courses of these drugs.

ANTIBIOTICS

If the patient has an infection, such as an abscess that is actually only a boil derived from the intestine, and caused by bacteria that live in the intestine, it is obvious that antibiotics should be used. If the patient is sick and the antibiotics do not work by mouth, they are given by vein. For this situation the drugs used usually include Ampicillin, tetracycline, Garamycin, and clindamycin.

Another antibiotic widely tried in Crohn's disease, especially in patients who have abscesses around the rectum or have had abscesses that started in the rectum and then reached through to penetrate the skin surrounding the rectum (known as fistulae), is metronidazole, better known to the public as Flagyl. Many women will recognize the name because it is used for the vaginal infection caused by trichomonas. There has been a flurry of concern about Flagyl because of its presumed cancer-causing effects, based mainly on mutation experiments on bacteria in test tube situations. I don't believe this is an important reason for not trying these drugs, if your doctor thinks it may help those nasty perirectal fistulae abscesses in your Crohn's disease. The real side effects to look for are those that cause neurological symptoms, mainly a neuritis—burning or numbness of fingers and toes. This symptom usually gives way when one stops the drug or reduces the dosage. In some cases the healing of Crohn's disease in the rectal area is remarkable.

IMMUNOSUPPRESSANT DRUGS

The newest group of drugs used in IBD is immunosuppressants, drugs that depress the body's immune system, that is, the system by which the body rejects foreign tissues. They were first introduced to prevent the body's rejection of transplanted kidneys. For about 15 years now they have been used to treat cases of IBD on the theory that the body was trying to reject its own tissues, and that these are actually, in fact, autoimmune diseases. The theory and success rate of these drugs in IBD remain controversial. They are widely used at present, especially in Crohn's disease, since doctors and patients wish to try any reasonable medical route before surgery. Whether their usefulness really depends on their immune suppressant activity or on their antiinflammatory activity remains unknown. Some very good results have been reported in patients who did not respond to the other medicines we use nowadays, but immunosuppressants take 6–8 weeks before they begin to take hold. If used carefully, which means repeatedly watching the patient's blood counts and reactions to other infections, they are safe, and their side effects are acceptable in a selected group. As far as I know, no tumors have been seen in patients with IBD treated with one of these medicines, either azathioprine, known as Imuran, or 6-mercaptopurine, known as Purinethol. None have developed any malignancies, but of course they have not been used routinely for a very long time.

Symptomatic Drugs

Since patients with IBD have cramps, intestinal spasm, diarrhea and, at times, abdominal pain, a variety of medicines are used to make them more comfortable while the antiinflammatory drugs (just discussed) are used at the same time. For the diarrhea and abdominal cramps caused by spasm, a wide number of antispasmodic pills are frequently given patients. These include Donnatol (a mixture of phenobarbitol and belladonna), Librax or Pathibamate (a combination of a mild tranquilizer and antispasmodic), and some antispasmodics that act on the smooth muscle cells of the gut directly (such as Bentyl). Many drugs have been used to slow down diarrhea. Most of these act by contracting the intestines so that the contents move through much more slowly and the number of bowel movements is decreased. The greater number are derivatives of opium or contain codeine (paregoric, deodorized tincture of opium) and their synthetic variants (Lomotil or loperamide). You must avoid acquiring dependence on them, and taking too many may cause a paralysis of the bowel. It is often difficult to decide what is causing the patient's pain, and you must not be given painkillers, which mask the situation. Also, doctors must take care not to make patients dependent on them. Patients are usually given mild pain relievers such as aspirin, Tylenol, or Darvon. Often stronger analgesics (pain-relieving pills), are required, especially codeine (which also controls diarrhea) and other opium derivatives. Quieting down the inflammatory process is the best way of handling the pain of inflammation.

Lifestyle

I said earlier in this chapter that anything that was good for you was also good for your intestines. The discovery that someone is suffering from Crohn's disease or ulcerative colitis should lead all concerned (the sufferer and the family) to take a good hard look at how the patient has been taking care of himself or herself. Has their way of life been as careful and wise as it ought to be? Just as business executives review their investment portfolios, patients must review their health portfolios and decide on future investments likely to improve their position.

Let us begin with habits. The restrictions on alcohol, tobacco, and caffeine have already been stressed. I have outlined what is reasonable to do about the diet. Equally important are the circumstances of eating this diet. Mealtimes should be regular. Schoolchildren must get up early enough to eat breakfast before running off to catch the school bus. The businessperson must not skip lunch in the press of work. If you are having lunch at your desk, shut the door and turn off the telephone. Patients with IBD who are well enough to go to work, and most can and do, need a small oasis of peace and quiet during the midday. We all have a limited amount of energy, some more, some less, but the laws of thermodynamics apply to us all as well as to the rest of the universe. Just as our checkbook must balance, so must our energy budget balance or we will be in the red. We can't spend more energy than we have. Patients least of all can afford to waste this energy.

Work, rest, and play are equally important. No doctor can write a prescription for the proper mixture, but you must not get overtired and overfatigued. You must encourage yourself or the patient to be active within the limitations set by the disease. Easier said than done.

Exercise is important both for its general effect on the patients' health and because it is a good outlet for the everyday tensions created by life within the family. Certain commonsensical rules should be followed. For the young patients, contact sports that run the risk of injury to the abdomen should be avoided. Patients should stop playing or exercising well before fatigue sets in. Those being treated with steroids should avoid sports that are likely to lead to broken bones. Other exercise that strengthens the muscles is worthwhile and necessary when on this group of medicines.

Games and sports should be played and enjoyed for their fun. I would discourage the stress that results from competitive games. The parents of young patients find it particularly hard to avoid being overly solicitous in this area. Guidelines of the kinds of sports and the amounts of time spent on them should be laid down firmly, but doctors and parents must not spend too much time hovering over children and patients. Having fun is important, as I have noted in the paragraph above. I do not believe with Norman Cousins in *The Anatomy of an Illness* that one can laugh away Crohn's disease or ulcerative colitis as he has reported with his rheumatological disorder. But having fun is important in sustaining the patient through the rough periods of this disease until recovery sets in.

Psychological Factors

Although you and your doctor do not know why inflammatory diseases happened to you, everybody's grandmother and next-door neighbor knows that colitis comes from nerves. I don't know whether disturbances of the patient's unconscious life lead to IBD, but I do believe that emotional turmoil and stress, both physical and psychological, can have a bad effect on the patient and his or her illness. Of course this is true of other diseases as well: tuberculosis, rheumatoid arthritis, and coronary artery disease, with or without heart failure, to name a few. In my observations, more psychological factors appear to be at work in patients with ulcerative colitis than in the those with Crohn's disease, but the key word here is *appear*. On the surface the patient with ulcerative colitis seems more sensitive and the psychological defenses weaker. Other observers are not convinced about this point, however, and stress the part that depression plays in Crohn's disease.

It is not difficult to see how an illness like Crohn's, occurring at critical times in the life of young people, can be a heavy burden to bear. Furthermore, even though we don't know all the factors causing IBD, it doesn't mean that we should not attempt to treat those disorders. Some cures were discovered long before the causes of the diseases were identified—quinine for malaria and liver extract for anemia are good examples. This question is not one you can settle theoretically; the real question is, does psychotherapy cure the disease? If it does not cure the disease and its attendant psychological stress, does it help?

I am not convinced that formal psychoanalysis carried out over long periods of time by rigorous analysts has cured my patients. I think a more helpful approach is to consult with a well-trained psychotherapist interested in IBD, if you and your doctor sense or suspect that your reactions to the many problems of living with the disorder may play a part in your symptoms and the continuance of disease. Psychotherapy and especially counseling may help you to come to terms with the fact that you have the handicap of disease. Emphasis on how to handle the problems the disease creates in your education, work, relationship with boyfriend, girlfriend, or spouse, helps to improve the quality of life, but I caution you not to expect miraculous results and then to fall into despondency and despair if "cure" does not occur. Everyone, especially those with these illnesses, needs to have or to learn ways of handling tension in a constructive fashion. Tranquilizers, in my opinion, except in the very short run, do not work. More potent and complex psychotropic drugs, mood elevators, "happy pills," require use by a skilled practitioner who prescribes them on a daily basis. Relaxation techniques, either by exercise, yoga, TM, music, or psychotherapy, are all different approaches to the same problem. You the patient must play a major role in making the decision to use them.

What Are the Results of Medical Treatment?

It's important to keep in mind the goal of treatment for you, your children, or other members of your family who have IBD. Of course you want to feel better, and go about your work and play, and hope that you will be "cured" of the diseases.

But "cure" is difficult. In *ulcerative colitis* the only known "cure" is to remove the colon surgically by an operation known as an colectomy. You and the doctor want to avoid this if at all possible. Remission to a normal condition *can* occur under modern medical therapy in this disease, with the colon returning to an absolutely normal state, and of course this is what you want and for as long as possible. Statistics on individuals who were never hospitalized for ulcerative colitis are sketchy, but of those who are hospitalized, at least two-thirds to three-fourths go into remission and can and do remain well for a long time.

The outlook for remaining well once you go into remission is improved considerably by staying on sulfasalazine for periods of up to 2–4 years. The dose for maintaining preventative treatment is smaller than the treatment dosage, and perhaps the newer, soon-to-be-released forms of 5 ASA (the active part of sulfasalazine) will allow you to take fewer pills and with the same or better protection. However, you must remember that feeling well and having no symptoms should not lead you to be careless. You will need to be under surveillance by your doctor because of the long-term risk of cancer in ulcerative colitis. I shall discuss how you can avoid this possibility later in this section.

Crohn's disease is a harder nut to crack, yet many people recover from it without even knowing that they had it, and a good number of people improve without medication simply by taking better care of themselves. Whether preventative treatment with medicine helps prevent return of sickness is far from proven, but if you are in remission and feel better, no matter how you got there, I think it would be reasonable to continue the same program. Salazopyrine or perhaps the new forms now being developed are reasonable medicines to stay on. Cortisone and the immunosuppressant drugs are riskier, and I'm not keen about them for preventing the return of symptoms.

All in all, the best information we have today says that for both diseases there is very little reduction in your expected life span, although there are going to be ups and downs along the way.

Frequently Asked Questions About IBD

What About Operations?

We would all like to avoid an operation, even the most trivial, for there are no trivial operations.

The possibility always remains, however, that our medicine may not do the trick, and that you may have to face the possibility of surgical treatment for either ulcerative colitis or Crohn's disease.

A few words on terms seem in order here.

A *resection of intestine* is the simple removal of part of either the small or large bowel or both, in which the normal cut ends of the tract are sewn together and the normal continuity of the intestine is kept.

An *ostomy* is an opening in the intestine; if in the small intestine or ileum, it is called an *ileostomy,* if in the large bowel, it is called a *colostomy.* Colostomies are usually performed on the colon to treat cancer of the rectum and not ulcerative colitis. If the colon must be removed to treat any form of colitis, an ileostomy will be performed instead.

Intestinal resections are performed most often for Crohn's disease of the small intestine, especially the ileum. Colostomies are usually not done for IBD. The possibility of an ileostomy following removal of the colon for any form of IBD exists for both ulcerative colitis and Crohn's disease.

Although the postoperative care and management of an ostomy of either the ileum or the colon is beyond the scope of this book, vou may want to consult self-help manuals and the ileostomy societies, which have meetings and visiting committees to acquaint patients with ways to live with an ostomy. Most modern hospitals caring for patients with IBD have trained therapists, called enterostomal therapists, to instruct the patient with the details of taking care.

What needs to be stressed here is that life with an ostomy can be carried on in a perfectly normal way. An ostomy poses no problems in dressing, bathing, swimming—none for almost all normal behavior. Indeed, dietary restrictions are few and far between.

It should be added that newer, more cosmetically acceptable operations for ulcerative colitis are being developed, studied, and performed at present. One is the Kock pouch, or continent ileostomy, in which a reservoir is fashioned from intestine. The other operation now unter intensive development is the pelvic pouch, in which the rectum is preserved.

In Crohn's disease, the modern surgical tendency is to remove as little of the intestine as possible, performing plastic surgery on the tight scarred areas that no longer allow food to pass through.

What Are the Results of Operations for IBD?

Since almost half of patients with Crohn's disease and perhaps a quarter of those with ulcerative colitis who are hospitalized have an operation some time in the course of their illness, this question is an important one.

For ulcerative colitis the answer is a resounding one: cure of the illness—but the price is one of the standard ileostomies or the newer cosmetic operations. You might ask then why not do an operation for all patients with ulcerative colitis? Although surgery does cure the disease, the majority of patients do not require an operation, and respond to the medical therapies already described.

For Crohn's disease the answer is a good one also, but perhaps not as resounding as for ulcerative colitis. In my personal experience more than 95% of Crohn's disease patients who have had an operation feel better, lead better lives, and would accept the operation again and recommend it to other patients. So why the hesitancy in Crohn's disease by both patient and doctor to accept this point of view? The possibility of recurrence, of course.

Although patients with Crohn's may have microscopic inflammation in their tissues or even abnormalities on x-ray after surgery, any clinical recurrence with sickness is much milder than the original disease and can be managed with medicines. Few patients require more than one operation. Occasionally, years after the original surgery, some patients may undergo reoperation to remove a narrowed, scarred area.

Although the risks of recurrence of Crohn's following operation are real, the liberation from dietary restrictions, freedom from pain and bleeding, and getting off the powerful drugs, make surgery attractive, especially if your symptoms are not responding to present medical treatment.

One bit of information about the timing of an operation is worth mentioning. The longer the patient has "waited out" the disease, the better the chances of staying well afterward. But the trick is not to wait too long. Here the judgment of your doctor and your own sense of whether you have made any progress toward getting better are important.

What About the Risk of Cancer?

Everyone runs the risk of cancer of the colon, which is the second most common cancer in males and the third most common in females. Although I discuss ways of avoiding and minimizing these risks in Chapter 4, here I want to discuss only the risks that come from having IBD, especially ulcerative colitis. By now everyone knows that the chances of having a cancer of the colon in this disease are greater than in the general population or by pure ill luck. But what are the facts?

First, cancer in IBD contributes only a small number of colorectal cancers in general.

Second, the risk is greatest in those with the disease in the whole colon, less in those with the disease in only a part of the colon, and least in those who have the disease in the rectum (the "proctitis" discussed earlier in this chapter).

Third, your age, whether you are female or male, and whether your disease is inactive or has made you sick for long periods of time, seems to make no difference.

Fourth, the most important point is how long you have had the colitis. The risk of trouble begins after you have had the disease for more than 10 years, and the chances increase about 1% each year after that. I have never seen a cancer occur in someone who had colitis for less than 9 years.

These being the facts, what can you do about cancer of the colon?

First, do not become careless because your colitis has not been bothering you for years. You are still at risk.

Second, remember whatever you may read in the literature or in the popular press, no doctor I know of advocates removing the colon from someone in good health just because he or she runs the risk of developing cancer.

Third, and most important, you must be under surveillance on a regular basis after you have had the disease, however quiet it may be, after the ninth year, because we now know how to prevent the development of cancer in the colon.

What Is Involved in the Surveillance You Need?

The colon must be inspected at regular intervals by colonoscopy. In this procedure a very narrow flexible instrument is introduced into the rectum and passed through the whole large bowel to the right side (the cecum). Done by an experienced physician, and following careful preparation so that your colon is clear of stool, and with some sedation given beforehand, this is a well-tolerated test. Although the risk is minimal, there is a possibility of bleeding or perforation; however, these are risks that a prudent patient should be prepared to take. This examination allows the entire lining to be scrutinized so that biopsies can be taken from any suspicious area. If none are seen, many biopsies can be taken from the entire length of the whole colon. The tissues are then examined for the earliest signs of a malignant tendency. These cellular changes are called *dysplasia* and signal trouble ahead. Good pathologists can distinguish dysplasia from mere inflammation. If dysplasia is found, you will be re-examined in 3 months to see whether it was the result only of inflammation, or confused with inflammation. If dysplasia persists to any marked degree, your colon must be removed to prevent the development of a cancer.

If the colon looks normal upon inspection, then you should simply continue to be watched because the odds are great against any small cancer being present.

How often will you need to be under surveillance? No one knows for certain, but I favor once a year or at least every 18 months, because a small cancer probably takes about 2 years to double in size. For this same reason, intervals shorter than 1 year don't seem practical to me.

With this kind of careful watching the risk of cancer can be tremendously reduced. There is also a growing feeling among the experts that doctors perhaps have been more concerned about the cancer problem in ulcerative colitis than incidence of the problem warrants. For the time being, however, I prefer doctor and patient both to be safe rather than sorry.

What About Crohn's Disease and Cancer?

Cancer in the small intestine is extremely rare. Although patients with Crohn's disease of the ileum have developed cancer there, they are relatively few—perhaps no more than 50 have been reported in the entire world literature since 1932. Cancer of the colon can and does occur in Crohn's, but to a much lesser degree than in ulcerative colitis. My hunch is that if you have Crohn's disease of the colon, you really don't tolerate the disease long enough to develop a cancer.

Why not take out everybody's colon after 10 years of IBD? Nobody wants a colectomy unless it's needed, especially if one isn't sick. The operation is a serious one and requires a permanent ileostomy, and, furthermore, Crohn's disease can come back. For all these reasons, I do not advocate operating merely to prevent a future cancer. Although no cancer of the colon is a good one, the risk on the whole is relatively small, and even smaller in the surveillance described previously.

We may need to change our minds the next 5 years as more evidence is collected, but, for the time being, colonoscopy with biopsies at fixed intervals is the best preventive plan to follow.

What About Members of My Family: Are They at Risk for IBD?

IBD is not a "catching disease"; very few family members have "caught" these diseases from their spouse, parent, or sibling. In some families, however, more than one member has the disease. The most common coincidence is mother and child, followed by siblings, with father and child the least likely. The occurrence of IBD in two family members does not prove that it is inherited, however. The coincidence might be due to common exposure to the cause or to a common susceptibility to the disease. IBD is not inherited in any simple, specific Mendelian way, the way hemophilia, for example, or other inherited diseases are passed from one generation to the next. If one of a pair of identical twins has IBD, the other need not have it also. Next, Crohn's disease and ulcerative colitis are not "Jewish diseases," although Jews do seem to have more than their share, so perhaps the susceptibility is inherited.

The important thing to remember is that no one can predict whether other members of your family will contract IBD. Certainly the decision of whether to have children should not be made solely on this point.

Can I Have Children?

If you are a woman with IBD who does not have a family, or wants to have more children, the answer is yes.

Unless you are so sick that you have lost a tremendous amount of weight and, like ballet dancers or marathon runners, do not ovulate or menstruate, you are as fertile as your neighbor who does not have this illness. IBD is not a contraceptive. Your chances of having a normal pregnancy and a normal child or a miscarriage are like those of well women.

You will feel better during your pregnancy if you're in good condition, especially when you conceive, if you've been stable or in remission for at least 6–12 months. Indeed, most women with IBD feel better during pregnancy, even if not at the onset, mainly because the placenta and the fetus provide additional cortisone. However, don't rely on pregnancy as a treatment for IBD!

Your pregnancy should be managed like any other woman's. You will not need a cesarean section just because of this illness, your prior history, including operations (even an ileostomy), and you should be allowed to deliver vaginally if you're able to do so. The only factor to take into consideration is whether you've had a lot of perirectal abscesses and fistulas with Crohn's disease. If so, this may influence your obstetrician's decision about a vaginal delivery or an episiotomy.

Delivery can be upsetting physically as well as emotionally, and sometimes patients have a little flare-up of their diseases afterward. If you can, plan on having more nursing and household help for you and the baby than you might have had without the disease, or following previous deliveries before you had the illness.

A frequent question that comes up in relation to pregnancy is what to do about medicines you are taking that are helping maintain your remission. Here intuition as well as facts play a part in my advice. There is a large and growing body of facts and opinions that supports the idea that drugs commonly used to treat IBD, salazopyrine and steroids, have no bad effect on the baby if the mother is taking them during the first trimester. All, however, agree that no woman on azathioprine or 6 mercaptopurine should be allowed to conceive. If at all possible, women should be taken off those drugs at the time of conception.

If, however, you become sick during the pregnancy, you can and should be treated with all the standard medicine used when you were not pregnant. My own and countless other physicians' experience is that these drugs do not have a bad effect on the baby.

The question of nursing the baby comes up all the time. Most doctors working in the field of gastroenterology see no problem if the mother is on steroids or salazopyrine. I tend to be more anxious and wonder whether a mother who needs these medicines should be allowed to nurse her baby, for her own sake, if not for the baby's. Certainly immunosuppressants should not be taken by a nursing mother.

What About Male Fertility?

Now for the male's problem. In general, men with Crohn's disease or ulcerative colitis do not have much difficulty in impregnating their spouses. The debilitating effect of IBD can reduce the sperm count, however, and make conception more difficult. In addition, one important fact has come to light in recent years: Salazopyrine can reduce the sperm count and thus diminish a man's chances of getting his partner pregnant. Although the drug has been used since 1946, it is only in the last few years that this effect has become quite clear. Still, many men on the drug can impregnate their partners. Equally important, the effect of salazopyrine on the sperm disappears quickly once the drug is stopped. Perhaps the newer form of the active principle (5 ASA) may reduce this risk. There is no evidence that prednisone or salazopyrine taken by the father has any bad consequences on the fetus. The immunosuppressants have not been used long enough to treat these illnesses to let us make any real predictions.

How Can I Better Care for Myself After Medical or Surgical Treatment?

Although ulcerative colitis can be "cured" by removing the colon, most patients keep their colon and thus face the possibility of a recurrence. The harder problem of treating Crohn's disease I have already discussed, mainly the problem of recurrences even after surgery.

Assuming you are now in remission—as a result of medical therapy in ulcerative colitis, and medical and surgical therapy in Crohn's—what can you do that will help you to stay well?

My first maxim is "anything that is good for you will be good for your gut!" Even without knowing the cause of IBD, it's obvious that physical and psychologic strain don't do patients with any disease any good.

I know of no dietary precaution that will prevent recurrences. If you are intolerant of lactose, you know this already. Obvious irritants of the intestinal tract in some patients, such as spicy seasonings, caffeine, and alcohol, clearly should be avoided. The major precaution is to avoid food fetishes and your next-door neighbor's advice regarding "bad foods." A well-balanced diet rich in protein with the accessory food factors (the vitamins) is what you need. Remember that while on salazopyrine your need for folic acid, a blood-forming vitamin, is increased, so that you'll need to take at least 1 milligram daily if your multivitamin does not contain this amount of "folate." If you have a narrowed area or "stricture" of the small or large intestine, obviously you need to chew food thoroughly and avoid roughage that can get stuck: Corn is a notorious offender, and unchewed mushroom or broccoli stems can also block the narrowed areas. If you are in a diarrheal phase, it's prudent to reduce the work of your intestine by reducing your intake of raw fruits and raw vegetables. For some reason, ripe bananas seem to slip by.

What about medication to prevent flare-ups? If you have ulcerative colitis, maintaining yourself on reasonable doses of salazopyrine, if you tolerate it, will reduce the chance of a flare-up or make the flare-ups milder and thus easier to treat. The new forms of this drug now under study may be even more protective since it will be possible to prescribe larger, more tolerable doses.

Salazopyrine taken by Crohn's disease patients in remission does not seem to affect their future health. Yet if you have had frequent flare-ups, and if you have had a recurrence soon after an operation, I would be inclined to keep you on salazopyrine, or perhaps the newer drug 5 ASA (when it becomes available) in an effort to minimize flare-ups.

This whole discussion should be seen in light of the fact that whether you have Crohn's disease or ulcerative colitis, once you go into remission you have a very good chance of staying well for long periods of time, even without any medication.

4

Diarrhea, Constipation, and Rectal Bleeding

Definitions

My definitions are quite simple. By *diarrhea* I mean bowel movements that occur too often and that are too loose. By *constipation* I mean difficulty in moving one's bowels. (Although some people think they are constipated if their bowel movements are dry and hard, these are not necessarily signs of constipation; again, difficulty in moving one's bowel is the important symptom.) By *rectal bleeding* I mean blood you can see with the naked eye on the toilet tissue, mixed with the stool, in the bowl, or all three. (Hidden bleeding, which doctors call "occult" bleeding, is blood in the stool that requires testing to be discovered.) Sometimes the stools may appear black, like older telephone models, or tarry in consistency. These symptoms are caused by stomach bleeding, which the action of intestinal bacteria turns black and sticky. Some stomach bleeding is so profuse that the blood does not have time to undergo a change in color. In this case, the blood remains bright red as it rushes down the whole intestine.

To put the definitions of diarrhea and constipation in proper perspective, the number of bowel movements that normal people in good health pass can vary tremendously, ranging from two or three per day to two or three per week. However, perfectly normal individuals may have many fewer or many more bowel movements than these average numbers.

Acute Diarrhea—"Intestinal Virus"

From time to time we all suffer episodes of gastrointestinal upsets in which we are nauseated, vomit, and have diarrhea. We cannot recall a specific meal or food that might have caused this episode; other members of our family may have similar discomfort. We are not part of an epidemic "going around," nor one of a group of people who went to the same banquet or picnic. The upset is usually mild, occasionally more severe; many times we have some fever with it, lots of loose stools sometimes with mucus, not often with blood. We are quite uncomfortable, but the whole illness is usually over in 3 or 4 days. We may not even call our doctor; we have had them before; we are prepared to wait this one out. If asked what was wrong with us, we pass it off as "an intestinal virus."

This kind of illness is the second most common clinical sickness in our society. Babies as well as adults have it, and traveler's from industrialized countries visiting developing countries are especially susceptible. This group of traveler's diarrhea deserves special attention. But stay-at-homes also get it.

What Causes Common Episodes of Gastrointestinal Upsets?

The infectious agents responsible for most acute episodes of gastroenteritis, whether viruses, bacteria, or parasites, are spread mainly by food or water contaminated by persons, animals, or the environment, and by person-to-person contact.

The viruses attack infants and babies and are mainly of the Rota virus group or the Norwalk agent. In adults the bacteria include *E. coli,* which produces a toxin, but the majority are bacteria of the *Salmonella, Shigella, Yersinia* entercolitica, and *Campylobacter* family. In the case of the last named, a sick household pet, such as a puppy, is frequently the source of the infection.

What Laboratory Tests Are Necessary to Diagnose Episodes of Acute Diarrheal Diseases?

For most individuals and most episodes of the mild varieties, no specific laboratory tests are required because no specific treatment is needed. You will recover by yourself.

In the case of the more severe forms, a simple test to confirm the diagnosis is to have the stool looked at for pus cells. If they are present, it will point to *Shigella, Salmonella, Campylobacter,* and occasionally *Yersinia.*

If you are sick enough to be hospitalized, are dehydrated, or have profuse diarrhea with fever, if the illness is going on for more than a week, and if you passed blood, then the stool should be cultured for abnormal bacteria, because you will need antibiotic treatment.

What About Treatment for Acute Episodes?

For most individuals with acute diarrhea, the illness is self-limited; you get over it by yourself. For the more severe or prolonged instances, replacement of the fluid and the electrolytes you have lost is essential; by mouth if you can take fluids, by vein if you cannot. For symptomatic relief, three main groups of medicines are frequently prescribed: (1) bismuth subsalicylate (in the United States in the form of Pepto-Bismol), which cuts down the secretion of the intestines but turns the stools black; (2) loperamide (Imodium) or diphenoxylate (Lomotil), which slow down the movements of the intestine and their secretions, but may worsen the disease by retarding the evacuation of the organisms responsible; (3) nonabsorbable earth mixtures of kaolin and pectin (in the United States Kaopectate). The latter are harmless and make the stools more bulky, but probably do little else.

Of the bacterial causes, most cases of *Salmonella* are not treated with antibiotics unless your bloodstream has been involved, then ampicillin is the drug of choice. For the others (*E. coli, Shigella, Campylobacter,* etc.), antibiotics of the sulfa group, especially the mixture trimethoprim/sulfamethoxazole (Bactrim, Septra) or erythromycin are in order.

The viral forms are rarely demonstrated by laboratory methods; for them we have no specific medicines and, except in the case of the dehydrated infant, they need no hospitalization or intravenous fluids.

What About Prevention of Sporadic Cases of "Intestinal Viruses"?

First, most of these attacks are not due to viruses. Second, since they are sporadic and you cannot predict when you will have an episode, or even whether you will have one, there is no safe preventative antibiotic medicine unless you are going to a developing country. We shall address ourselves and this specifically in the section on traveler's diarrhea.

What About Food Poisoning?

We only think about an episode of food poisoning when more than one individual experiences the same illness shortly after partaking of the same food. They are mostly caused by some of the bacteria already mentioned earlier in this section and by toxins produced by bacterial organisms. In many instances, the specific agent is not found or identified for technical reasons, or because the suspected foods are no longer available for testing.

One may suspect that a particular organism has caused the outbreak, because it is associated with some common foods that are prone to carry the organisms. A list of these is given in Table 4.1.

TABLE 4.1 Common Food-Borne Illnesses

Carrier	Organism
Beef	Salmonella Staph. aureus
Ham/pork	Salmonella
Poultry	Salmonella Campylobacter Staph. aureus
Eggs	Salmonella Staph. aureus
Cheese	E. coli Salmonella
Fish/shellfish	Clostridium botulinum Vibrio cholerae Salmonella
Fried rice	Bacillus cereus

Traveler's Diarrhea

Nowadays millions of people travel all about the world and run the risk of developing *traveler's diarrhea* (T.D.). By this we mean having at least twice the usual number of stools and having them loose. Most of us have experienced this in one or more forms. Usually the attack begins abruptly while abroad or soon after we get home. You may experience abdominal cramps, nausea, bloating, the need to empty your bowels in a hurry, a general sick feeling, and a fever. Rarely, the diarrhea may be violent and accompanied by rectal bleeding. Most people get over traveler's diarrhea rapidly by themselves.

Ordinary T.D. causes four to five loose watery stools per day and may last 3 to 4 days; only 10% of the time does it last longer than 1 week. So if you have a chronic case of diarrhea after returning from travel abroad, it may be different from the ordinary garden variety of T.D. Very few deaths can be attributed to traveler's diarrhea.

Who Gets Traveler's Diarrhea?

Your destination is the most important factor in determining whether you will get traveler's diarrhea. People from a developed country visiting a developing country run the highest risk, but even in the least developed countries perhaps only half of all travelers get a diarrheal disorder. The highest-risk destinations are the developing nations of Latin America, Africa, the Middle East, and Asia. Lower-risk destinations include most of southern Europe and a few Caribbean islands, excluding Haiti and the Dominican Republic. Those areas and regions in which one is least likely to get traveler's diarrhea include Canada, northern Europe, Australia, New Zealand, the United States, and Caribbean islands not included in the preceding risk category (see Table 4.2).

Curiously, young adults seem to develop traveler's diarrhea slightly more often than older adults. The reason may be that young people are often more adventurous in their style of travel and try new and different foods. For all travelers, raw foods, including raw vegetables, raw meat, and raw seafood, are expecially risky. Tap water, tap water ice, unpasteurized milk and dairy products, and unpeeled fruit can also cause T.D. Where you eat is also very important: Street-vendor food carries the greatest risk of causing T.D., with restaurant food somewhat less risky, and food served at private homes posing the lowest risk. The important point is that traveler's diarrhea is acquired through eating food or drinking water that is contaminated with fecal material. Even cooked food, if handled improperly, may carry the causative infectious agent.

What Causes Traveler's Diarrhea?

T.D. is caused by infectious agents: bacteria, viruses and, rarely, parasites.

All travelers who enter a developing nation from a developed one, and who have consumed local food and drink, undergo a quick change in their intestinal flora, the organisms that ordinarily inhabit the intestinal tract. Those who get T.D. have ingested a

TABLE 4.2 Areas of Risk for Travelers' Diarrhea

Low-risk Area	Moderate or Unknown Risk Area	High-risk Area
Australia	Albania	Afghanistan
Austria	Argentina	Africa (all countries ex-
Belgium	Bulgaria	cept South Africa)
Canada	Caribbean Islands	Bangladesh
Denmark	(other than Haiti	Burma
Finland	and Dominican	Cambodia
France	Rep.)	Central America (all
Germany (East and	Chile	countries)
West)	China	Dominican Republic
Ireland	Cuba	Haiti
Isle of Man	Cyprus	India
Japan	Czechoslovakia	Indonesia
Liechtenstein	Greece	Iran
Luxembourg	Greenland	Iraq
Monaco	Hong Kong	Korea
Netherlands	Hungary	Laos
New Zealand	Iceland	Mexico
Norway	Italy	Nepal
South Africa	Israel	New Guinea
Sweden	Jordan	Pakistan
Switzerland	Pacific Islands	Philippines
United Kingdom	Poland	Saudi Arabia
United States	Portugal	South America (all
	Romania	countries)
	Spain	Sri Lanka
	Taiwan	Syria
	Tasmania	Thailand
	Union of Soviet So-	Turkey
	cialist Republics	Viet Nam
	(Russia)	
	Yugoslavia	

Source: Herbert L. DuPont, M.D. and Margaret W. DuPont, M.A. *Travel with Health.* New York: Appleton Century-Crofts, 1981.

sufficiently large dose of the infectious agents for their normal gastrointestinal defense system to be overcome.

The commonest bacteria are the *E. coli*. These release a toxin that causes the bowel to pour out large amounts of secretions, especially fluids and the electrolytic ions of the blood, which, in turn, lead to dehydration. Other bacteria include *Salmonella, Shigella*, and *Campylobacter*. A group of viruses (*Rotavirus* and *Norwalk*-like virus) may also cause T.D.

Despite what you might expect, parasites do not often cause T.D. Those that can cause T.D. are amoeba and the parasite *Giardia lamblia*. Most travelers have heard of the large outbreaks of giardiasis in Switzerland, Leningrad, and Aspen, Colorado, in recent years.

Very often no organism—whether bacterial, viral, or parasitic—can be found, or may be sought too long after the attack has begun to be detected.

How Can I Avoid Getting Traveler's Diarrhea?

At present and probably for some years to come, there are no vaccines for the organisms that cause T.D. Thus, care in the preparation of food and beverages, and meticulous attention to where and what you eat and drink are the best preventive measures. The use of Lomotil (diphenoxylate) or Imodium (loperamide) does not prevent T.D., although most travelers carry and use them. However, bismuth subsalicylate (the active ingredient of Pepto-Bismol) taken in the liquid form (2 ounces four times a day) has prevented some travelers from developing T.D. But taking large doses of bismuth subsalicylate for 2- to 3-week periods on a trip not only means taking a huge supply with you, but may be risky. Most doctors advise against it and so do I.

A few antibiotics, such as doxycycline (Vibramycin) and trimethoprim/sulfamethoxazole (Bactrim, Septra), taken as a precautionary measure, can reduce the chances of developing T.D. However, their side effects, including the form of colitis associated with antibiotics, lead me to advise against their preventative use. Their other side effects include common skin rashes, sensitivity to sunlight, bowel disorders, and fungal infections of the vagina. The risks are just too great to hand out these drugs to all travelers who might develop T.D.

What Treatment Works in Traveler's Diarrhea?

Although for most travelers T.D. is a nuisance and not a serious illness, we all want relief from cramps and diarrhea. A large number of popular remedies have been used over the years to "absorb" the toxic agents of T.D. (activated charcoal, for example) but they don't work. Kaolin and pectin (Kaopectate) give the stools a firmer consistency, but otherwise do not help a lot.

Drugs against diarrhea that work by slowing down the bowel include paregoric and opiates, which have been long used, and the newer synthetic agents (Lomotil [diphenoxylate] and Imodium [loperamide]). These drugs can give temporary symptomatic comfort but should not be used if the symptoms continue for more than a few days. Travelers should remember that Pepto-Bismol turns the stool black (and that the change in color is not due to blood) and that aspirin should be avoided while taking it, because both in conjunction can irritate the stomach.

It is very important to replace the fluid (water) lost from the intestines from T.D. to avoid getting dehydrated. Milk and dairy products should especially be avoided. If you are mildly dehydrated, you ought to drink potable fruit juices, caffeine-free soft drinks, consommé, and safe water, and eat salty crackers. More dehydrated individuals may find solutions such as Gatorade, Lucozade, or mineral water with added sugar, useful. In the severe forms of T.D., which resemble cholera, you may need some mixtures of electrolytes in water, which can be taken by mouth or even intravenous fluids. You will need to consult a physician to obtain these.

If you are sicker than most travelers with nausea, vomiting, fever, severe abdominal pain, or even bloody stools, antibiotics can help shorten the illness. The sulfa drug, trimethoprim, or the combination sulfas (Bactrim, Spectra) for no more than 3 or 5 days are useful.

In all of these situations, care must be taken if the individual is a child or a pregnant woman. Kaolin and pectin are harmless, but try to get by without the others if you are pregnant. Tetracycline can stain the teeth of children under 12, and the sulfa combinations may cause a skin rash and sensitivity to sunlight at all ages.

Parasites

T.D. is a self-limited, short, acute illness, and is rarely caused by parasites. If, however, you have persistent diarrhea after returning home from abroad, it's important to have a test for parasites and some bacteria in the stool. This means culturing the stool for *Campylobacter* (a "bug" that hangs on), and looking for the two commonest parasites in the freshly passed stool—*Entamoeba hystolytica* (the cause of amebiasis) and *Giardia lamblia,* which often has the upper abdominal symptom of nausea and indigestion as well as diarrhea. Sometimes an antibiotic taken for T.D. can itself cause a diarrheal disorder (almost all antibiotics have been shown to be able to cause this), and the laboratory must look for the toxin of *Claustridum difficile* in the stool as well. If it is present, it can be handled in several simple ways.

As you finish this section, you might wonder whether you ought to travel at all, but this would be the wrong conclusion. For most travelers, T.D. is a short, self-limited nuisance, not a major medical hassle. Some elementary care in what and where you eat and drink will protect most people, and simple remedies or none at all are the best treatment.

Other Forms of Diarrhea

To understand diarrhea, you should know that the movement of fluid through the intestines is a big deal. The stomach, liver, gallbladder, and pancreas pour many quarts of water into the gut. The small intestine absorbs most of this fluid as it moves downstream, so that only 1–2 pints (500–1000 cc.) enter the colon. On the right side (see Figure 1.1) the stool is compacted and dehydrated so that normally only 3 to 6 ounces (100–200 cc.) of water escapes with the stool. Only a slight interference with this orderly process can cause the colon to be overwhelmed by the fluid load, and this gives rise to diarrhea. Any disturbance in the colon that interferes with compaction, storage, and drying of the stool will further increase the likelihood of diarrhea.

Acute Diarrhea

Most episodes of acute diarrhea, of which traveler's diarrhea is a good example, are due to an infectious agent, the most common being viral. Sometimes the virus or bacteria is not present in the infected food we eat, but the product of this virus or bacteria— their toxins—is. *Staphylococci* are frequent causes of outbreaks of diarrhea among members of a picnic, for example, who have eaten a custard pie or poorly refrigerated foods, and all come down with diarrhea. The family of *E. coli,* which produces the irritating toxin discussed earlier under "Traveler's Diarrhea," is usually the most frequent cause of this type of diarrhea. *Shigella* or *Salmonella* are other kinds of bacteria that cause acute diarrheal diseases. Recently, there have been reports of outbreaks of diarrhea due to contamination of milk with *E. coli* during the course of pasteurization. An outbreak of diarrhea among those who ate a commercially available cheese infected with *Listeria monocytogenes* was also recently reported in the Midwest.

These forms of acute diarrhea are self-limited: You get over them by yourself in a short time, and they require no specific treatment, except the replacement of the salts and water lost with the diarrhea (discussed in detail under "Traveler's Diarrhea"). More intense or unusual forms require culture of the stools and search for *amoeba* or *Giardia*. Bleeding during these episodes of acute diarrhea raises the possibility that the attack may be the beginning of a more serious illness, such as ulcerative colitis or even Crohn's disease (although bleeding is less common in Crohn's).

With acute, self-limited forms of diarrhea, you should be careful not to take too much of the drugs that slow down the diarrhea. Lomotil and Imodium are the most frequently prescribed today in the United States, but may prolong the illness. Still, their judicious use is helpful, as are the innocuous Kaopectate (kaolin and pectin mixture) types.

Chronic Diarrhea

The more persistent forms of diarrhea are more annoying, upsetting, and difficult to diagnose and treat because they can be confused with the irritable bowel syndrome (discussed in Chapter 2).

Gastric-Colic Reflex Diarrhea

By some individuals, having too many formed stools is considered diarrhea. Often these bowel movements cluster around the conclusion of a meal   breakfast being a very common offender—when the sufferer must race off to the bathroom as soon as his or her meal is finished. The food just eaten has not rushed from the stomach to the rectum in such a short time, but rather the meal has triggered off the *gastro-colic reflex,* a reflex in which neural and chemical messengers released from the intestine signal the colon to empty itself. Sometimes this may be due to lactose intolerance but, more frequently, it represents a hyperactive nervous system. Drugs that slow down the transmission of such reflexes may be helpful if taken before meals. These are most often medicines of the belladonna or atropine group and are currently available in pill forms of varying dosages, which need to be adjusted to each individual's needs.

Secretory Diarrhea, Malabsorption Syndromes, and Parasites

More difficult to sort out are the true chronic diarrheas. Some are insidious and annoying, not always active, cause a low-grade sickness, and are due to parasites. More serious forms are associated with weight loss, which signals that the intestine is failing to absorb the calories we eat and, hence, are known as *malabsorption syndromes*. There are others in which the loose stools occur by night as well as by day or even if no food has been consumed; these are due to the intestine secreting excessive amounts of fluid and are thus called *secretory diarrheas*.

PARASITES

Even in the United States, and even if the patient is not very sick, it is important to have the stools examined for parasites in the milder form of chronic diarrhea. *Entamoeba hystolytica* and *Giardia lamblia* can be difficult to find, so the search must be very diligent. One does not have to go to the tropics to pick up these organisms; in this sense even New York City can be considered a tropical isle. Giardiasis is notorious in certain parts of the world, and epidemics have originated in Aspen, Colorado, Zermatt, Switzerland, and Leningrad in the U.S.S.R. The secret to finding parasites is to examine fresh stools, preferably passed in the laboratory or brought directly from home and examined before they dry out. It may require several examinations, at least up to three, to exclude amebiasis, the infection with ameba, although a special blood test may help point the way to this diagnosis. Smears of the stool taken directly through a sigmoidoscope may reveal the organism if stained appropriately. *Giardia lamblia,* which often causes some nausea along with the diarrhea, is quite elusive because it lives in the upper intestine in the duodenum and thus may not be seen in the stool specimens. In the search for these culprits, it may be necessary to obtain juice from your duodenum by passing a tube through the mouth to that area. On rare occasions, both of these organisms may be found embedded in the tissues of the duodenum or colon only when biopsies of these places are done and a specific search made for them.

Tedious as the search for these parasites may be for patient and doctor, it is clearly worth the effort since eliminating these chronic "boarders" in the intestine by modern combinations of drugs will cure the condition.

SECRETORY DIARRHEAS

Some forms of chronic diarrhea have nothing to do with eating but are due to fluid secreted by the intestine, the so-called *secretory diarrheas.* These may be caused by small, often hidden tumors, especially in the pancreas, which release chemical messengers that stimulate the bowel to pour out vast amounts of liquid.

Because the volume of water lost from the intestine in this kind of diarrhea mimics cholera, it has been labeled "pancreatic cholera." The secretory diarrheas are difficult to diagnose because the tumors are often tiny. A combination of screening techniques and blood and urine tests for their messengers, the hormones, help to locate the cause, however.

Because secretory diarrheas are quite rare and those caused by tumors are among the rarest, it's important to remember that certain medications can mimic their symptoms. The drugs that most commonly cause secretory diarrhea, and that are often the hardest to detect, are laxatives and "water pills" (diuretics). These are hard to detect because individuals often take them secretly, usually in a desperate attempt to lose weight. These instances are quite rare, too, but more frequent than the tumors.

But what about the "harmless" things we all eat? *Intolerance to lactose,* the sugar of milk (discussed in Chapter 2 on the irritable bowel) certainly can give some individuals frequent, loose stools. Beyond this, a whole list of foods are blamed by different people as the cause of their diarrhea. There certainly is biochemical individuality as there is personality individuality, but one must be careful about eliminating one food after another because of suspected "food intolerances" or "food allergies." From a statistical point of view, milk, eggs, and wheat are the most likely offenders. Some people also have a limited ability to digest and absorb starch as well, and there are curious interactions between starches and wheat. You ought to avoid developing lopsided diets by eliminating one food after another without some proof that these foods really are causing your chronic diarrhea. Here, the guidance of a doctor is especially important.

MALABSORPTION

If our intestine fails to properly digest food and/or to absorb the products of digestion, then we lose calories, mainly in the form of fats, in the stool. This usually leads to larger, softer stools, and not always to diarrhea. These fatty stools have a light, oily appearance, are frothy, and are quite malodorous. They often float on the water in the toilet bowl. We used to think that this was because oil floats on water, but now we know it is due to gases trapped in the stool. With the loss of nutrients there follows the inevitable weight loss.

For malabsorption to be the main cause of weight loss, the individual must be eating an adequate diet. This is an important point. *Malnutrition* due to inadequate intake of food for whatever reason (bad appetite, poor dentures, aversion to food as in hepatitis) is not *malabsorption*. Weight loss is due mainly to the malabsorption of fats since they carry the bulk of our calories. On the other hand, if you are gaining or maintaining weight despite chronic diarrhea, it is most unlikely that you have *malabsorption*.

Symptoms. The diarrheas associated with malabsorption are marked by looser or loose stools. In addition, you may experience bloating, gas, abdominal distention, and the passage of malodorous gas through the rectum. These gases arise from the action of intestinal bacteria on the rancid, unabsorbed fats in the diet and their subsequent release in the form of gases such as methane or hydrogen sulfide (which has the smell of rotten eggs). Just as the amount of weight loss may vary tremendously, these symptoms may range in intensity from mild to very severe.

Diagnosis. Malabsorption has many causes and sorting them out is like solving a crossword puzzle or, better still, like putting together the pieces of a complicated jigsaw puzzle. Before undertaking a detailed search, your doctor first needs to document the malabsorption (this includes ruling out malnutrition). He or she will also need sound records of your previous weight to document how fast and exactly how much weight you have lost. Especially helpful is an exact record of your actual food intake on a daily basis. A carefully kept food diary (kinds, times, and amounts) will help enormously.

The first step is to collect evidence of failure to absorb fats. Blood counts and measurement of your blood for vitamin B_{12} and the factor called folic acid will show whether you are failing to absorb these materials, which are vital for making red blood cells properly filled with hemoglobin. If you are anemic (that is, your blood cells and stores of iron are low), your doctor must be sure that this is not due to a slow loss of blood from the intestine by repeated examination of your stool for hidden bleeding.

The next question is whether you are losing fat in the feces. A simple but crude way to find out is to have a specimen of the stool stained for fat and examined under a microscope. The most accurate way, however, is to eat a diet high in fat and to collect the stools for 24, 48, or, better still, 72 hours. This is messy and tedious, but it is the only reliable way to answer this question. Most of us absorb almost all the fat we eat (no wonder we gain weight if we don't watch out!) and waste only 7 grams (less than 2 ounces) each day in our bowel movements. People with real malabsorption may lose up to 20 or 30 grams per day or even more.

Some forms of malabsorption are caused by failure of the intestine to absorb the sugars (carbohydrates) in our diet. The simplest way to detect this kind of malabsorption is to do a d-xylose test. This sugar is taken by mouth and its level in the blood and urine measured after 5 hours of collection.

Once it has been determined that you have a malabsorption, the search for the cause begins in earnest. I shall not describe all the causes in detail, because the list is long and the causes may exist in the stomach and all along the intestine.

If your *stomach* has been operated upon for ulcer disease, for example, and the food stream has been rerouted, malabsorption may result. Trouble in the *liver* or improper functioning of the *gallbladder* or its removal may also, on occasion, interfere with the digestion and absorption of fats.

The *pancreas* is a key organ in digestion, especially in fat digestion. In children, cystic fibrosis of the pancreas, in adults, chronic inflammation of the pancreas can result in severe malabsorption.

Disease of the *small intestine* affects the lining cells, so that even properly digested foods can not be absorbed. Inflammation and tumors head the list here, with disorders of the ileum being the most serious.

In children as well as adults, a frequent and correctable form is *coeliac disease,* the inability to handle a specific protein—gluten—present in wheat, rye, oats, and barley (as in the old nursery rhyme!) and cured by a diet from which gluten has been rigorously removed.

If identification of the cause depends on detecting the exact nature of the tissue changes in the small intestine, it may be necessary to do a small bowel biopsy. This sounds worse than it really is. The patient swallows a very thin tube, which passes into the upper small intestine, where it takes a biopsy of the lining of the bowel. This is a safe procedure and often gives the exact information required to treat some forms of malabsorption, especially coeliac disease.

Constipation

The simplest definition of constipation is difficulty in moving one's bowels. More precisely, it is needing to strain to have a bowel movement more than 25% of the time. What is "normal" varies tremendously. Although normal individuals move their bowels between three times a day and three times a week, many others move theirs more or less frequently, some as seldom as every 3–5 or even 9 days, and some as often as three times a day.

We all may have short periods of "constipation," whatever definition we use. Accustomed to our own routine, we may have temporary difficulty on a trip or if we don't have access to our own bathrooms. But it is when this difficulty persists that we become uncomfortable and worry about its meaning, in part because doctors have alerted everyone to pay attention to any change in bowel habits in an effort to diagnose cancer of the colon at an earlier and more treatable stage. The main point to remember is that it's not the occurrence of a change that's important (we all may have a temporary change), but its persistence.

If you do experience persistent constipation, stop to consider whether you are taking any new medicines before you contact your doctor. A great many, especially those for the control of high blood pressure, can affect the motility of the colon. Other drugs that cause constipation include painkillers containing codeine, morphine, or opium in any form, antacid gels containing aluminum compounds, and many psychotropic drugs, such as the mood elevators and those used to treat parkinsonism. Iron by itself as a pill or in vitamin mixtures can cause the stool to become dark, almost black, induce cramps, and constipate some individuals. Medication-related constipation is easily remedied by stopping the medication (with the consent of your doctor), or having your doctor find a substitute drug without this annoying but harmless side effect. Another thing to consider is whether you have for some reason cut down the amount of fiber you are eating by reducing your intake of fruits, salad, unrefined vegetables, and cereal carbohydrates.

If neither medication nor a change in diet accounts for persistent or steadily increasing constipation, it's time to contact your doctor. Here, as in the irritable bowel syndrome, your history is very important: Some families have a predisposition to develop constipation; some patients have been taking a medication for so long that they have forgotten this fact; and, finally, the age of onset of constipation can also provide a clue as to whether the problem might be of the congenital forms of neurologically based constipations. The chief example of the latter is Hirschsprung's disease, which may show itself soon after birth or in the first few years of life. A person with this disorder lacks certain nerve cells in the lowermost segment of the rectum. This defect in the "wiring" of the rectum prevents the rectal and anal sphincters (the muscles that are the "doorkeepers" of the colon) from relaxing when the need arises for them to do so.

Your history also may bring out some general symptoms not directly related to the bowel problem, but which may be clues to a

general medical problem concerning the endocrine glands, hypothyroidism (inadequate or low function of the thyroid gland, for
example), or a metabolic problem such as too much calcium in the
blood (such as disorders of the parathyroid glands). Injuries to the
spinal cord or the spine can also affect the nervous control of one's
bowels. Difficulties of bowel function have also been noted following gynecologic operations such as hysterectomy. In some instances, disturbances in the bowel are associated with concomitant difficulties in emptying one's bladder. Here again the history taking is
the most important clue to the problem.

Only a carefully taken history will reveal whether psychological
factors (early toilet training, for example) or the symptoms of
depression, such as loss of appetite and sleeplessness, are part of a
general picture in which constipation is but one feature. You and
your doctor should also discuss whether you have suppressed or
disregarded the call to have a bowel movement because of place or
time. Habitual disregard for the urge to defecate can interrupt the
normal pattern, and calls for re-establishing the conditioned reflex.
Early in the history taking you should be prepared to discuss, frank-
ly and fully, whether, and to what extent, you have become dependent on laxatives, cathartics, and enemas (although the last is least
harmful).

Your doctor will want to know if you have noted any blood in
your stools. If so, this raises the question of whether the colon is
blocked by growths (benign or malignant). Your doctor will also
want to know whether you have any rectal pain, because he or she
will be looking for some local cause in the rectum which has inter-
fered with the usually painless act of defecation.

Finally, there are some rarer forms of constipation that are
related to more general disturbances in the muscles or nerves serv-
ing the entire gastrointestinal tract. In addition to difficulty in moving your bowels, you may experience difficulty in swallowing.
These peculiar forms of constipation are called "pseudo obstructions" because they mimic true mechanical obstructions and have a
curious associated symptom called Raynaud's phenomenon: a
change in the blood flow to the fingers which, as a result, cannot

tolerate cold and become blue or dead white in the cold or on picking up ice cubes, for example. At times, difficulty in emptying your bladder goes along with problems in the colon in these conditions.

What Tests Must I Undergo to Determine the Cause of My Constipation?

Aside from a general physical examination to see whether you have the signs of some endocrine disturbance, attention will focus on the lower bowel. Rectal examination with the finger and testing the stool for hidden bleeding are necessary routines. The rectum and anus will have to be looked at to be sure you have no local trouble, such as a fissure (a painful crack in the skin where the lining of the anus joins the external skin). Certainly a sigmoidoscopy is next in order. (Sigmoidoscopy sometimes may reveal patches of a brown pigment in the lining, so-called *melanosis coli* due to the prolonged use of cathartics that contain carcara, a popular laxative.) A barium enema after cleaning should also be done to determine whether you have been constipated so long that the colon has actually become enlarged; this is called a megacolon. Naturally any tumors would also be detected.

If it is suspected that you may have a more complex problem because of faulty nerve reaction in the rectum and anus (on a congenital basis, as in Hirschsprung's disease), pressure studies, the so-called *motility studies,* may need to be done. In these harmless and painless studies, a very thin tube is passed into the rectum, and the pressure on the tube is recorded on an oscilloscope. Sometimes it is useful to measure how slowly or rapidly things move through the intestinal tract. This measurement is called transit time. Performed by taking an x-ray of the intestine on successive days after you swallow some radio opaque (not radioactive) markers, this test not only can tell how fast or slowly the contents of the intestine are moving, but also whether the markers are held up at a specific place in the intestine.

What Are the Usual Causes of Constipation and How Are They Treated?

The commonest cause of constipation in the Western world is inadequate fiber and roughage in the diet. It has been clearly shown that in other parts of the world (Africa especially), where the native population lives on a diet high in unrefined vegetable carbohydrate, constipation, as well as the irritable bowel and even diverticular diseases and cancer of the colon, are much less frequently seen than in the developed countries of the West. As a result, current treatments of constipation call for a marked increase in dietary fiber in the form of certain vegetables, raw fruits, nuts, flour, and especially cereals. Tremendous emphasis has been given to taking bran and certain plant seeds, namely, psyllium seeds (which are the active parts of Metamucil and related products).

What Is Dietary Fiber?

Even experts have trouble defining this term. It includes all the complex plant carbohydrates that cannot be digested in the intestine by our digestive enzymes; this means all those substances that enter the colon undigested. In the normal small intestine, almost all food substances and most liquids and vitamins are completely absorbed, so only some water and its ionic components (salts of sodium and vitamins) and those undigestible residues of plant foodstuffs enter the colon. A small part of some starches (potato, rice, etc.) escape small bowel digestion as well.

Once fiber enters the colon, the local bacteria digest it, adding bulk to the stool and increasing its water and gas content by fermentation. Just how fiber does this is far from agreed upon. Formerly, it was thought that the increase in the bulk of the stool was due solely to the water-holding action of intact fiber, but this is not believed at present. It may be due to the stool's increased bacterial content since these intestinal organisms can and do live on fibrous materials. (Remember that half of the normal stool is made up of bacteria.) Fiber also hastens the transit time and lowers pressure in the lower colon, and perhaps this allows the contents to pass through more easily and faster.

Treatment with High-Fiber Diets

I highly recommend a high-fiber diet to those who are constipated and urge them to eat the raw fruits and raw vegetables listed in Table (4.3). In addition to fiber content, some foods, such as prunes and figs, contain naturally-occurring substances that stimulate intestinal evacuation. An old-fashioned plant laxative, senna, was used by our grandmothers and great-grandmothers in the form of a tea. (More recently, senna has been marketed in a standardized form, commercially known as Senokot).

The switch to a high-fiber diet is often hard for some people because their intestines need time to adjust to the new diet.

Working at the High-Fiber Diet

The first thing to do before starting the high-fiber diet is to make an inventory of what you are actually doing as far as fiber is concerned. You may be like many people. Because they eat some salad and fruit, they believe they are on a high-fiber diet. You will need to keep track of everything you eat over a 3-day period, listing the foods and a rough estimate of the amount. By referring to Table 4.3, you can make a calculation of the actual amount of fiber in your daily customary diet. For most individuals who really need lots of fiber, it is quite startling for them to find out that they are taking in very small amounts. Most of the experts in this field agree that you ought to aim for between 25–30 grams of fiber daily, and most of us don't consume anywhere near that amount.

You can see from Table 4.3 that meats, poultry, eggs, and dairy products contain absolutely no fiber, and many fruits have very little. (Strawberries and blackberries, curiously enough, have lots.) Green vegetables vary tremendously (from the very little in a cup of raw spinach to 3.5 grams in a half cup of broccoli). Breads and

TABLE 4.3 Dietary Fiber

	Amount	Weight (grams)	Fiber (grams)
Bread and crackers			
Graham crackers or digestive biscuits	2 squares	14.2	1.4
Pumpernickel bread	¾ slice	24	1.4
Rye bread	1 slice	25	.8
Whole-wheat or whole meal bread	1 slice	25	1.3
Whole-wheat cracker	6 crackers	19.8	2.2
Whole-wheat roll	¾ roll	21	1.2
Cereals			
All Bran, 100%	⅓ cup	28	8.4
Bran Chex	½ cup	21	4.1
Corn Bran	½ cup	21	4.4
Corn Flakes	¾ cup	21	2.6
Grape-nuts Flakes	⅔ cup	21	2.5
Grape-nuts	3 Tbsp.	21	2.7
Oatmeal	¾ pkg.	21	2.5
Shredded Wheat or Wheatabix	1 piece	21	2.8
Wheat flakes	¾ cup	21	2.6
Fruit			
Apple	½ large	83	2.0
Apricot	2	72	1.4
Banana	½ medium	54	1.5
Blackberries	¾ cup	108	6.7
Cantaloupe	1 cup	160	1.6
Cherries	10 large	68	1.1
Dates, dried	2	18	1.6
Figs, dried	1 medium	20	3.7
Grapes, white	10	50	0.5
Grapefruit	½	87	0.8
Honeydew melon	1 cup	170	1.5
Orange	1 small	78	1.6
Peach	1 medium	100	2.3
Pear	½ medium	82	2.0

(continued)

TABLE 4.3 *Continued*

	Amount	Weight (grams)	Fiber (grams)
Pineapple	½	78	0.8
Plum	3 small	85	1.8
Prunes, dried	2	15	2.4
Raisins or Sultanas	1½ tbsp.	14	1.0
Strawberries	1 cup	143	3.1
Tangerine	1 large	101	2.0
Watermelon	1 cup	160	1.4
Meat, Milk, Eggs			
Beef	1 oz.	28	0
Cheese	¾ oz.	21	0
Chicken/Turkey	1 oz.	28	0
Cold cuts, hot dogs	1 oz.	28	0
Eggs	3 large	99	0
Fish	2 oz.	56	0
Ice cream	1 oz.	28	0
Milk	1 cup	240	0
Pork	1 oz.	28	0
Yogurt	5 oz.	140	0
Rice			
Rice, brown (cooked)	⅓ cup	65	1.6
Rice, white (cooked)	⅓ cup	68	0.5
Leaf Vegetables			
Broccoli	½ cup	93	3.5
Brussels sprouts	½ cup	78	2.3
Cabbage	½ cup	85	2.1
Cauliflower	½ cup	90	1.6
Celery	½ cup	60	1.1
Lettuce	1 cup	55	0.8
Spinach, raw	1 cup	55	0.2
Turnip greens	½ cup	93	3.5
Root Vegetables			
Beets	½ cup	85	2.1
Carrots	½ cup	78	2.4
Potatoes, baked	½ medium	75	1.9

(continued)

TABLE 4.3 *Continued*

	Amount	Weight (grams)	Fiber (grams)
Radishes	½ cup	58	1.3
Sweet potatoes, baked	½ medium	75	2.1
Other Vegetables			
Beans, green	½ cup	64	2.1
Beans, string	½ cup	55	1.9
Cucumber	½ cup	70	1.1
Eggplant (Aubergine)	½ cup	100	2.5
Lentils, cooked	½ cup	100	3.7
Mushrooms	½ cup	35	0.9
Onions	½ cup	58	1.2
Tomatoes	1 small	100	1.5
Winter squash	½ cup	120	3.5
Zucchini squash (Courgette)	½ cup	65	2.0

Based on analyses of dietary fiber prepared by James W. Anderson, M.D., *Plant Fiber in Foods,* University of Kentucky Medical Center, 1980.

crackers do not have very much fiber content. The cereals, especially the brans, have the highest amounts.

Once you embark on a high-fiber diet, it will become clear to you that you are going to have to work at it to achieve the desired amount in your daily intake. It is not easy; eating in restaurants and fast-food shops until recently also presented obstacles, but now that the value of the high-fiber diet in reducing a whole host of disorders has become better known in our society, salad bars and vegetable platters have been multiplying. But still it will not be easy until increasing your intake becomes an automatic habit.

In addition to the plant seed supplements to your diet, another way of getting enough fiber into your daily food intake is to use some fiber cookies. Several kinds are conveniently available; Fiber Med and Fiber Rich are just two of the commercially available forms sold in drugstores and food shops. These contain about 5 grams of fiber in each cracker and are rather palatable. My simple rule is to add one new substance at each meal and to slow down if you get unpleasant signals from your intestine, such as rumbling, gas, or even discomfort. But don't give up; stay with it, and your bowels will adjust.

More About Bran

Bran, the raw natural milled form, often called Miller's bran, is a very good source of fiber, and 1 ounce can give you quite a lot. A simple way to take it is to add it to your usual cereal, shake it into cottage cheese, or mix it with yogurt. Individuals vary and some cannot tolerate much or even small amounts of bran. If, after a real try, you find you are one of these people, then give up trying bran; the other forms of fiber will do just as well. For those of us who cannot tolerate bran, the psyllium seed preparations are excellent substitutes. There are a number of such preparations easily available; probably the best known is Metamucil, which comes either in bulk packages or small individual packets. These preparations are not too unpalatable and should be taken with water, or they can be blended with fruit juices. A convenient time to take them is before going to bed. As with all medicine, the dose must be adjusted for each individual.

What About Lubricants?

Lubricants, of which mineral oil is the best known and the longest used, are not absorbed in the intestine and thus supply "oil" to the intestinal tract, where they lubricate the hard stool in the colon of the chronically constipated person. Nowadays, lubricants are frowned on because they are habit forming, may interfere with the absorption of certain vitamins (those that dissolve in fat), and may be inhaled into the lungs, especially in youngsters.

A more acceptable form of lubricant, sodium dioctyl sulfate, is sold by prescription in the form of Colace or can be bought over the counter as Surfak. One does not want to become dependent on these substances, but they are harmless.

For those individuals who have lost the sensations that remind us to defecate, or whose awareness of those sensations has been blunted by years of constipation, only the use of laxatives, sometimes in combination with a simple, nonmedicated suppository, which restores rectal sensation, may do the trick. The use of suppositories that depend on irritating chemicals (Dulcolax, for example) should be avoided except on rare, isolated occasions. (They are of the type used in preparing the colon for x-ray examination.)

What About Enemas?

Although it's not a good idea to become dependent on artificial stimulation to start off a bowel movement, of all the local stimulants a simple tap water enema—distending the rectum with warm tap water instilled by means of a baby bulb syringe—is certainly the most harmless. This kind of enema mimics the natural distension of the rectum by the stool, and sets off the reflex by which the rectum empties itself as the "trap door" muscles or sphincters open themselves.

Fluid Intake

Many people misunderstand the affect of liquids in the diet on bowel movements. In a healthy state, the body's requirements for fluids are closely regulated by thirst. If you satisfy your thirst and your kidneys are normal, you will take in enough water and put out enough urine. Remember that the fluid content of your diet cannot wash out the colon, because the small bowel absorbs most of the liquid you drink and only a small amount enters the colon. Ordinarily the small intestine absorbs water so efficiently that even a slight disturbance, caused by illness, for example, can overwhelm the colon's ability to handle the fluid load. Attempts to liquify hard, dry stools by increased fluid intake rarely work unless your "normal" intake of fluid in all forms (milk, tea, coffee, soups, water, soft drinks, etc.) has been grossly deficient.

Lifestyle

Normally, having a bowel movement doesn't require any thought: It is an automatic act based upon a conditioned reflex. When having a bowel movement becomes a problem, we try to recondition our bowel habits by restoring that conditioned reflex. It may help to try to defecate every morning at the same fixed hour, perhaps after breakfast, taking enough time. For some, a cup of coffee may be enough of the stimulant to set off the reflex; for others, reading a newspaper and thus distracting the mind may help.

Good general muscle tone is important because the contractions of the diaphragm and abdominal muscles are part of the complex act of defecation, and weak muscles cannot do the job. I advise all patients who suffer constipation to do regular physical exercises involving the abdominal muscles. Runners and joggers have usually discovered for themselves that these exercises often trigger a bowel movement.

Rarer Forms of Constipation

Poor diet, poor toilet habits, and the hurry and stress of urban life are the most frequent causes of constipation. We have come to recognize in recent years, however, that these factors do not explain every case; some rarer forms of constipation are caused by diseases.

Hirschsprung's Disease

The best known of these rare types is Hirschsprung's disease. This form is due to a fault in the neural connections in the wall of the lower bowel, usually in the rectal segment. As a result, one portion of this segment is narrowed and contracted and fails to open up normally. The disease occurs full blown in the earliest years of life and causes marked constipation. If it's not recognized, it may cause the colon to dilate tremendously and become what is called a *megacolon.*

Some milder forms of this disorder may not be easily recognized and may go on in a low-grade form for many years, masquerading as the common form of constipation. Indeed, the oldest person I have seen with this disorder was 59.

One of the most important clues to this disease is whether you have had trouble moving your bowels from infancy. If your parents are alive, their history of your early bowel habits can be very important in tracking this down. If there is an early history of constipation or your colon is becoming much bigger than usual, your doctor will need to pursue this diagnosis further.

WHAT ARE THE TESTS FOR HIRSCHSPRUNG'S DISEASE?

The simplest test is a barium enema, but without the colonic cleansing out needed for other disorders. This so-called unprepared barium enema may show the narrow, contracted segment mentioned above. The findings of the barium enema need to be confirmed by motility studies of the rectal segment (described earlier in this chapter), which will show whether the rectal sphincter relaxes when the colon is stimulated by a small balloon. Failure of the sphincter to relax further suggests that Hirschsprung's disease is present.

The final step in making a diagnosis is to perform a biopsy of the tissues of the rectum. These are stained in the laboratory for nerve cells. These nerve cells (ganglion cells) are missing or reduced in number, and special stains may need to be done. Since the results of operation for this condition are so good, it is worthwhile having these tests done if there is a reasonable chance that you have some form of Hirschsprung's disease.

Other Rare Disorders

Even rarer, but capable of causing a lot of distress for the individual and confusion and difficulty for the doctor, is a group of curious disorders of the entire intestinal tract. In recent years these have been called "pseudo obstructions." People who suffer from these disorders have trouble not only in moving their bowels but in swallowing or emptying their bladders. They often act as if they had a mechanical blockage of their intestine, and may be operated upon only to have the surgeon discover that there is no obstruction. These rare forms may be familial or congenital (from birth). When the intestine is biopsied, it may show evidence of a prior viral infection or degeneration of intestinal muscle or intestinal nerves.

Rectal Bleeding

In this section I want to discuss the general subject of rectal bleeding, and will talk only about the blood that is visible to the naked eye. Rectal bleeding that is associated with specific diseases is covered in the sections of each disease.

The closer to the rectum that bleeding arises, the brighter red the blood. Bleeding from hemorrhoids, which are often associated with constipation, may appear on the toilet tissue, as a streak along a formed stool, or may be passed purely as blood into the bowl. In colonic disease, rectal bleeding may be mixed with the stool. Blood arising further back in the colon may be maroon or as dark as port wine, but it will not be black. The blood may also be mixed with mucus (the clear, jellylike fluid that the colon pours out as a lubricant). This mucus may clot and turn white or brown, and patients may mistake this for a worm or think they are passing tissue from the wall of the intestine.

All Rectal Bleeding Should Be Taken Seriously But Need Not Be Due to a Serious Cause

Anytime you have rectal bleeding, you should report it to your doctor, who must consider it in the light of what he or she knows about your general condition. I believe every episode of rectal bleeding must be investigated.

What Are the Essential Steps in Investigating Rectal Bleeding?

As always, a good history of the circumstances is the key: Your recent travel history and your recent history of medication are part of this inventory.

On physical examination, your doctor will note whether you are pale, sweaty, or have low blood pressure. These are clues to the fact that you have lost a lot of blood quickly. In addition, he or she will have a blood count done to determine whether you are anemic or have been bleeding for some time unbeknownst to you. Your doctor will, of course, do a rectal examination, attempt to obtain some stool from the rectum, and test it for blood. The rectum must also be examined by an anoscope to see whether you have internal as well as external hemorrhoids. Your lower bowel must also be looked at directly as far as the sigmoid (see Figure 1.2) by sigmoid-oscopy.

Even if these examinations appear to identify the source of the blood, the remainder of the colon should be examined to be sure there are no other possible causes of rectal bleeding. For this purpose, x-ray of the colon, the barium enema described earlier (page 20), is the best method. If this test does not find the cause, and the x-ray of the upper intestinal tract, the GI series, and the small bowel x-rays (described on page 36) also reveal nothing, then a colon-oscope examination of the entire colon is called for.

You may think that this is a lot of examination, unpleasant preparation, and expense for a little bit of blood, but the stakes are high. It is crucial to determine that you do not have a dangerous or potentially dangerous source of bleeding, such as a polyp or a cancer.

In most cases, this series of tests will reveal the source of the bleeding. Causes may range from the innocent to the malignant: internal and/or external hemorrhoids, inflammatory bowel condition (ulcerative proctitis or colitis or variations of Crohn's disease), polyps of all sorts with differing malignant potential, curious vascular anomalies (mainly on the right side of the colon and seen with a colonoscopy), infectious diseases (viral, bacterial or parasitic), and diverticular disease (to be discussed in Chapter 5), and a variety of malignant tumors.

In these few cases in which these tests do not provide an answer, your doctor may continue to observe you. Indeed, if bleeding persists, there is no alternative. This means continuing to examine the stools for obvious or hidden blood and to measure the hemoglobin and red blood cell count of the blood. Although some doctors may want to repeat the x-rays, many feel that repeating the endoscopic examination (especially colonoscopy) may be more revealing. This should be done by another observer who may have better luck or skill, but not necessarily.

When the bleeding is not immediately visible, the search for a cause can become tedious and time-consuming, since the source may be anywhere along the entire intestinal tract. The longer the bleeding continues without any obvious source becoming apparent, the more likely is the chance that the cause is benign and not malignant.

Small benign tumors of the small intestine and lesions of blood vessels of the small intestine are the hardest to locate. In these situations, other techniques may be required. A very useful one is a special scan in which your red blood cells are labeled with a tracer, reinjected into your veins, and your abdomen scanned periodically for hours. This may reveal the site and even the source of bleeding, but may have to be repeated many times to be sure. More rarely, it may be necessary to do an angiogram (an x-ray of the major blood vessels of the abdomen similar to the better-known blood vessel x-rays of the heart, the coronary angiogram); however, this necessity is rather rare. The common causes of rectal bleeding are the ones most often found. The moral is clear: The source of the bleeding may be trivial, but the search for the source must be serious.

Even More About Fiber

Since there is so much interest in fiber at present (and I predict we will continue to be even more concerned in the future), I want to add a little more for those who are interested. Many terms are used for this class of plant materials that are not digested by the secretions of the human intestinal tract: unavailable carbohydrates, non-nutritive fiber, edible fiber. Dietary fiber remains, in my opinion, the most useful label.

The chemical constituents of these plant fibrous materials need not concern us here. Known as celluloses, hemicelluloses, pectins, and lignins, these are all present in the tissues of vegetables and fruits, apple peels, peanut skins, and especially cereals.

These dietary fibers have a great water-holding capacity: 100 grams of turnip fiber will hold 1 ounce of water, while 100 grams of bran fiber will hold up to 15 ounces of water. They affect the rate at which materials pass through the intestinal tract from stomach to rectum, increase the bulk of our stools, and bind bile and the products of fat digestion. We are just beginning to learn what they do to the whole range of intestinal digestion and absorptive functions.

Fiber in our diet can interfere with the enzymes that digest fat especially by "tying" them up, so to speak, thus decreasing the amount of fat that can be absorbed. The result is a loss of fat and cholesterol in the stool and a lowering of their amounts in the blood. This is clearly the case with oat bran, but corn bran and beans probably act in different ways in reducing blood cholesterol. So you see why, in our current attempts to reduce heart attacks by reducing blood fats and cholesterol, the emphasis on fiber is so important. These fibers do this also by binding the parts of the bile that are needed to dissolve the fats before they can be digested and then absorbed. This whole area further reinforces our need to take in a goodly amount of "roughage" not only for our bowel's sake, but also for our heart's sake.

Although we cannot digest the complex carbohydrates of the dietary fibers, the bacteria in the colon can. Some of this digestion may be useful to us by releasing constituents of mucus, which could replenish the protective, jellylike coating of the colon. On the other hand, the bacteria can release gases in the colon, which result from the process of fermentation. So you can appreciate why the effects of dietary fiber on the action of intestinal bacteria are being studied so intensively at present, especially their possible part in preventing tumors of the colon by preventing bacteria from altering the bile salts that do reach the colon.

Not only the fats of our blood but our blood sugars as well can be lowered by the dietary fiber we eat. Carbohydrates taken in fiber meals produce a lower blood sugar, lower than when eaten without fiber and, in diabetic persons, fiber lessens their requirements for insulin. This seems to be due to the effect of fiber in slowing stomach emptying and also slowing intestinal absorption of sugar as well. Interestingly enough, a fiber meal at breakfast has a carryover effect, lowering sugars taken at lunchtime. Even more interesting, kidney beans, red lentils, and soybeans (called as a group legumes) are better for us in this regard than bread, rice, or potato.

5

Polyps and Cancer of the Colon

We all live with the fear of developing a cancer; in men, cancer of the colon is now the second commonest cancer in the body; in women, it may soon become the second commonest also. In both sexes, colon cancer is by far the most common cancer of the entire intestinal tract. In this chapter, I use the term *colon cancer* to mean any cancer that develops in the colon from the cecum to the rectum, instead of continually saying colorectal cancer. Where there are important differences between cancer in the rectum and cancers elsewhere in the remainder of the colon, I make that difference clear. There is nothing good about cancer of the colon, but of all the gastrointestinal cancers, including those in the esophagus, stomach, pancreas, liver, and biliary system (gallbladder and bile ducts), colon cancer has the best outlook for cure and survival of life. If cancer of the colon is detected early and promptly removed by operation, you have better than 85–95% chance of cure.

The key to prevention of colon cancer is the link between polyps and cancer. Polyps (which will be discussed later in greater detail) are benign growths, but they can turn malignant. All current research leads to the uncontestable conclusion that polyps are the precursors of cancers: Eradicate the polyp and we can prevent its development into cancer.

Causes of Cancer of the Colon

Fifty years of intensive research has convinced those working in the field that human cancers are the result of a variety of factors, different in each kind: a mixture of genetic and environmental causes. The problem is even more complex since the incidence of different kinds of cancers varies around the world and the various incidences are changing.

That heredity plays some part in gastrointestinal cancer is obvious. There are some families that are cancer prone. The Bonapartes had a great tendency toward cancer of the stomach. The condition known as familial polyposis of the colon is inherited in strict Mendelian fashion and invariably leads to colon cancer if not removed surgically. Modern molecular biology has begun to dissect out the specific genetic patterns that involve the so-called *oncogenes*.

Whatever the future may discover, the genetic factors are of course not under our control at present. So the focus at present in gastrointestinal cancer is on the search for environmental factors, and investigators look for trends. Cancer of the stomach in the United States, for example, has been falling steadily since 1980. No one knows why for certain, but the cleanliness of our foods has improved, and I suspect that reduction in frying everything in brown fat has also played a role. It is certainly reasonable to think that, as in the link between cancer of the lung and smoking, there are some things we are taking into our bodies that might be involved in intestinal cancer.

It must be significant that although the incidence of cancer of the colon is low in Japanese at home, when they emigrate to the United States, their incidence of colon cancer rises along with the rise that is occurring in cancer of the colon in U.S. natives.

In some instinctive way we all feel that the environmental factors that trigger genetically susceptible individuals to develop cancer of the colon must be taken into our bodies in our food and diet, so many studies have focused on the link between diet and colonic cancer. Although this relationship is still being researched, two factors figure prominently in most of these studies: diets high in animal fats and low in cereals, fruits, and grain (that is, low fiber and/or low-residue diets) seem to be associated with colonic cancer. Whether these are two separate factors, or whether people (especially in developed nations) who eat larger amounts of animal fat also have diets that are relatively low in grains and cereals and fruit is not clear. It has been speculated that it is the interaction of bile salts secreted by the liver, the fatty acids derived from the partially digested animals fats and intestinal bacteria, which is intimately involved in setting off the malignant process in the lining cells of the colon.

Even if the association between high animal fat/low-fiber diet and colonic malignancy has not been proven, it is worth bearing in mind. Reducing the amount of animal fat and increasing the amount of cereal, fruit, and grain in one's diet is prudent for this and other very good reasons, including the need to reduce fat and cholesterol intake to prevent or reduce the risk of heart disease and heart attacks. I have been impressed by how many of my patients on their own have reduced their intake of red meat and baked foods prepared with butter and eggs, and now use skim milk or low-fat cottage cheese. Influenced generally by information offered in the press for laypeople, they feel better for these changes in their dietary habits. The reduction in death from heart disease for example, which began in the United States even before the newer medical and surgical treatments became widespread, can be credited to these dietary changes.

Cancer in the intestinal tract occurs mainly in the two storage areas—the stomach and the colon—where food or food residues remain in contact with the lining for longer periods of time than in the small intestine. This is another reason why a high-fiber and increased vegetable diet, which will empty out the colon frequently, is a reasonable one to follow. Because we know so little about other aspects of diet and colonic cancer, however, it would not be wise to avoid other foods simply because you suspect they may increase your chance of getting cancer; you may develop a lopsided diet as a result. Recently it has been suggested that the calcium in our diet may play a protective role in preventing cancer of the colon. When the overactive intestinal cells of certain colonic cancer-prone individuals were studied in the laboratory after these individuals were given calcium supplements of 1½ times their usual daily recommended requirements of 700 milligrams, the cells "quieted down" and behaved more like a normal individual's colon cells. Perhaps by the time you read this more evidence will be available to guide us in deciding how useful calcium supplements will be in preventing colonic cancer.

Although cigarette smoking has thus far not been linked to colonic cancer, it has been associated with cancer of another part of the gastrointestinal tract, the pancreas. (This cancer has also been increasing in recent years.) For this reason among many others, it is prudent to stop smoking cigarettes.

In its authoritative report, *Diet, Nutrition and Cancer* (National Academy Press, Washington, DC, 1982, pp. 400–401), the Committee on Diet, Nutrition and Cancer of the National Research Council summarizes this problem:

> . . . three hypotheses appear to be supported by various strengths obtained from epidemiological studies of both colon and rectal cancer: (1) a causal association with total, and perhaps saturated, fat; (2) a protective effect of dietary fiber; and (3) a protective effect of cruciferous vegetables (green leafy vegetables, broccoli, cabbage, brussels sprouts, and yellow vegetables such as squash).

Although some studies have raised the question of whether alcohol plays a role in causing rectal cancer, this is far from proven and requires further study.

Polyps

The importance of colonic polyps for the prevention of cancer bears repeating: *Eliminate the polyp and you eliminate its becoming a cancer.* Hardly anyone in the United States now does not know about the search for President Reagan's polyps.

A polyp is a benign, yet nonetheless abnormal, growth. You may have heard that smokers can develop polyps on the vocal cords from exposure to the irritating smoke of cigarettes, or that opera singers can develop them from straining their voices. Allergic individuals can have them in the nasal passages and women can have them in the vagina or in the womb.

These growths occur on the linings of the body and are made up of the different cells that compose the linings. Polyps that develop from the tissue lining the colon, which is called the *mucosa,* are made up of the glands that line the surface and secrete the protective slimy mucus that acts as a lubricant for material coming down the colon.

True Polyps

The polyps that are precursors of colon cancer are known as *true polyps.* A word you may hear applied to them is *adenoma,* which simply means a glandular polyp. Their appearance under the microscope varies; some resemble small tubes ("tubular polyps"), others look like seaweed with waving fronds ("villous polyps"), and some contain features of both types ("mixed polyps"). It was once thought that villous polyps had a greater tendency to become cancers, but this has since been disproven. All true polyps should be removed.

Although an x-ray of the colon (Figure 5.1) or an endoscopic examination does not reveal whether a polyp is malignant, they do show its shape, which can be an important clue. If the polyp is on a stalk (Figure 5.2), like a grape on a stem, it is more likely to be benign. If it's resting flat on the surface ("sessile"), it is more likely to contain malignant cells (Figure 5.3). Because the tip of an other-

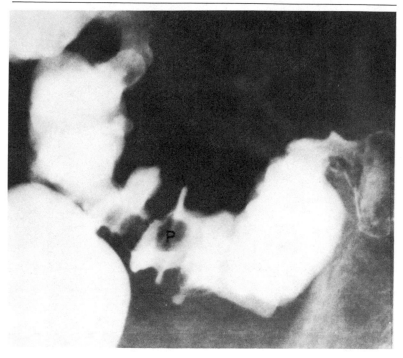

FIGURE 5.1 Polyp of colon on a stalk seen on barium enema. P = polyp.

wise benign-looking polyp on a long stalk can contain malignant cells, however, the whole polyp must be removed and carefully examined by competent pathologists.

Inflammatory Polyps

Sometimes the heaped up tissue in the colon forms a tiny protuberance resembling a very small wart. These benign growths, known as *inflammatory polyps,* result from local inflammation of the wall of the colon. If your doctor detects them during sigmoidoscopy or colonoscopy, he or she will simply remove them and perform a biopsy to be sure that they're truly benign.

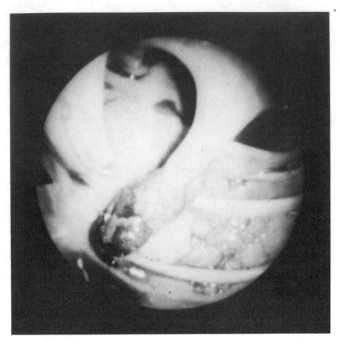

FIGURE 5.2 Polyp on stalk seen through the colonoscope.

Pseudopolyps

People with inflammatory bowel disease sometimes develop false or pseudopolyps. These are areas in the colon where the inflamed tissue has "heaped up." As seen by x-ray or endoscopic examination, these areas mimic true polyps but are not in fact growths as far as we know, and are not forerunners of cancer. Because individuals with any disease of the colon (including ulcerative colitis and Crohn's disease) can develop polyps, your doctor must take care to distinguish between pseudopolyps and true polyps.

The pseudopolyps do not in themselves present any medical problem, but are confusing because they can on x-ray resemble true polyps, and thus raise the question of whether they are potential

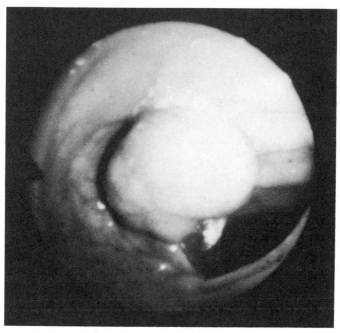

FIGURE 5.3 Polyp of the colon seen through the colonoscope. This "sessile" polyp sits directly on the inner lining of the colon.

sources of cancer. This is especially worrisome in a disease like ulcerative colitis, which has an increased incidence of cancer. Biopsy of these pseudopolyps will easily answer these questions.

Sigmoidoscopy or a limited flexible endoscopic examination can detect true polyps, but because the instruments used in these examinations do not reach all the way into the whole colon, a complete colonoscopy is needed to check for additional growths. Some doctors like to precede the colonoscopy with a barium enema x-ray, sometimes together with an x-ray of the remainder of the upper intestinal tract, so that they will have a good "road map" of your gastrointestinal system. This "map" will reveal whether you have any other disease of the colon or whether there are any obstacles, such as diverticular pockets, strictures, or scars, that may pose problems in the colonoscopy. Other doctors may just as reasonably prefer to forego this preliminary examination and perform a complete colonoscopy straightaway. During the colonoscopy, your doctor can biopsy the original polyp and any others seen along the way. Whether your doctor performs a barium enema x-ray and a colonoscopy, or just the latter, the goal is to determine whether your colon has polyps in addition to the original one and to biopsy any and all polyps that are encountered.

Symptoms of Polyps

Because colonic cancer usually starts as a polyp, searching for polyps is an important step in preventing its development. Polyps may show themselves by a change in bowel pattern, rectal bleeding, the passage of mucus from the rectum and, in a few cases, the passage of voluminous amounts of fluid from the rectum.

CHANGES IN BOWEL PATTERN

Although temporary changes in bowel movements due to infections or changes in toilet habits, food, or water are normal, changes that persist are not. How long you should wait before consulting your doctor is difficult to answer, but don't wait more than a week.

PASSAGE OF BLOOD OR/AND MUCUS WITH THE STOOL

Mucus, a clear or cloudy jellylike material, lubricates the colon. The passage of mucus with the stool can occur in the irritable bowel syndrome, but the passage of bloody mucus does not, and should alert you to have this looked into promptly. (Rectal bleeding is discussed more fully in Chapter 4.)

RECTAL PASSAGE OF LARGE AMOUNTS OF FLUID

Although this occurs most frequently in infectious diarrhea, in a few instances it is due to the *villous adenoma*. This type of polyp pours forth large amounts of watery fluid that contains all the fluid elements of the blood except the red blood cells. This in turn leads to the loss of many vital substances from the blood, especially potassium, and this in turn leads to muscle weakness.

Some polyps cause no symptoms and thus are extremely difficult to detect. If you belong to a family with a history of cancer and/or polyps, then your doctor probably already has you under surveillance. But what should you do if you have no family history of cancer or polyps?

Prevention

Beginning at age 40, it's a good idea to have a yearly physical examination, which includes a manual rectal examination. Most doctors now believe that one ought to have a sigmoidoscopy as part of the routine physical examination every 2 years. Although the rigid sigmoidoscopy (20 cm.–10 in.) and even the newer flexible fiberoptic sigmoidoscopic examination see only a portion of the whole colon, these examinations of the left side of the colon are worthwhile since more than half the colon polyps are in that portion.

Although some doctors advocate periodic colonoscopy, and a smaller number advise x-rays in the search for asymptomatic polyps before they cause trouble, these do not seem reasonable tests to have done every few years during one's adult life. Colonoscopy carries with it the risk of perforation of the colon, and barium enemas entail exposure to radiation. Nor do we have a simple blood test for the presence of a colonic polyp and none for colonic cancer.

For those with none of the symptoms I have already discussed in this chapter, our best approach at present is examine the stools for hidden blood, so-called occult bleeding.

Because of current concern that premalignant polyps and cancer of the colon be detected and treated early, great interest has been focused on testing the stools of people at risk for developing these conditions.

The most widely used test in the United States at present is the Hemoccult test. In this test a fragment of stool that has been retrieved from the toilet bowl is smeared on a strip of test paper. The strip has been impregnated with a substance (gum guaiac) that turns blue when a drop of a developer containing hydrogen peroxide is placed on it, if the stool contains blood. Another strip, which does contain blood and which reacts strongly to the developer turning dark blue, serves as a control for comparison.

A number of factors can influence the results of this test. First, the test does not distinguish between sources of blood, so a positive reading may result from blood from anywhere in the intestinal tract (including bleeding gums), not just the lower bowel and colon. Fortunately, blood originating high in the intestinal tract is less likely to be detected. Second, the test is not specific for human blood, so a person taking the test must avoid beef in any form, such as steak, roast beef, and beef hamburgers. Chicken, fish, pork, and veal, which contain little blood, do not seem to affect the test results.

Third, other foods, such as cantaloupe, grapefruit, and cucumbers, may mask the test. Although some studies insist on the subject taking a high-roughage–high-fiber diet, this has not been shown by careful testing to be necessary.

Fourth, a variety of drugs and other substances can also interfere: aspirin, iron, and vitamin C (ascorbic acid).

Given these various factors, it's clear that you must take care in doing the test to avoid a false positive (getting a blue color when it is not due to your own bleeding into the intestine) or a false negative (not getting a true blue color although your blood is in the intestine). The best way to prepare for taking the test is to adhere to the following dietary rules for at least *3 days before* collecting the stools and *during the entire period you are collecting them:* Avoid all red meat, cucumbers, cantaloupe, grapefruit, iron tablets, vitamin C tablets, and aspirin. You should collect six specimens (two separate portions of three different days' bowel movements) and mail them promptly to your doctor.

Sensitivity

Since this test is meant to detect the presence of blood hidden in the stool and does not directly test for the presence of polyps or colonic cancer, its sensitivity depends on how often and how much the polyps or cancer bleeds. Not all cancers, even ulcerated ones, bleed, and polyps may bleed even less than cancers. For this reason it is preferable to send in six specimens from *three different days,* not just three consecutive stools especially if passed on the same day.

Accuracy

In a mass screening of people for polyp, colon, and rectal cancer, the test accurately identified up to 66% of those subsequently proven to have malignancies. None of these people had symptoms at the time they were tested. Although further research is underway to determine whether individuals without symptoms should routinely use the test, regular testing under any of these circumstances does seem worthwhile:

- Your family has a history of cancer or polyps of the colon
- You are over the age of 40, so your doctor should do the test routinely as part of your annual physical checkup
- You have any bowel symptoms, such as change in bowel habits, or are anemic

If two sets of tests have positive results, a careful search for the cause of the bleeding is imperative. Remember that in the vast majority of people the cause is usually a trivial one—hemorrhoidal bleeding, for example. If the cause is not immediately apparent, however, the search may require other tests: a barium x-ray of the colon (barium enema) and, if this reveals nothing, x-rays of the remainder of the intestinal tract. If the source of bleeding still remains unclear, a colonoscopy of the lower bowel is in order.

Other Tests

Two other tests of blood in the stool have been or are being developed. One is *HemoQuant,* which detects hemoglobin and its degradation production by a fluorescent method. The test is very sensitive, but is relatively complex technically and is not yet commercially available on a routine basis.

Another test detects the human hemoglobin in the stool by immunochemical methods. Although it shows great promise, this approach needs to be simplified and tested before we know its full value.

Conclusion

Despite its limitations, the hemoccult test is worth doing because it is the best one we have to date, which can be used in a routine fashion.

Removing the Polyp

Removing a polyp that hangs in the colon by a stem is simple and has extremely few complications. (Perforation of the colon, the severest complication, is fortunately extremely rare. Bleeding may occasionally occur, but the endoscopist can easily control this.) Problems arise if the pathologist finds malignant cells in the polyp. If the cancerous cells are situated on the *surface* of the tip or of the whole polyp, but have not penetrated into the stalk, nothing more needs to be done at this time. If, however, the malignant cells have penetrated into the stalk, an operation on that segment of the colon from which the polyp arose is necessary. This allows the surgeon to remove the lymph glands that drain the area and to have them examined for spread of tumor cells. The surgeon will also check visually for spread of the cancer to the liver, although metastases are not necessarily visible to the naked eye.

Removal of flat sessile polyps presents a problem. Because they cannot easily be snipped out, many biopsies must be taken to be sure that they contain no cancerous cells. They can be removed piece by piece through the endoscope, but one cannot be sure that the whole polyp has been removed. As a result, a more formal abdominal operation is advised to insure that the whole polyp is removed.

If the polyp is big and flat and occupies the rectum, it is possible to avoid the drastic measure of removing the rectum by removing the tumor by fulguration (multiple, staged attacks in which the tumor is burned by electrical cauterization). But again in these polyps, it is imperative that each piece removed be examined for cancer.

Preventing Recurrences

While we have little knowledge of what causes polyps, how they become locally malignant, or how they can be completely transformed into a cancer, certain things we can do seem prudent. Eating a diet high in fiber and low in animal fat seems a sensible course to follow, and perhaps being sure one has an adequate calcium intake (Table 5-4); keeping the colon under surveillance by periodic stool and endoscopic examinations is another. (Careful examination of six stool specimens at 6-month intervals for hidden blood and an annual colonoscopy seem a reasonable timetable to follow, although we have no real scientific evidence on which to base these guidelines.)

No blood test at present can tell us whether a cancer is developing in the body. The CEA test (carcinoembryonic antigen) depends on finding a tumor marker in the blood when a large enough collection of colon cancer cells have spread beyond the wall of the colon into draining lymph nodes, and especially into the liver.

Familial Polyposis

Familial polyposis is a potentially fatal disorder which, as its name implies, is genetically transmitted. It usually appears in late adolescence (ages 15–20) and almost always by early adulthood. A person with this disorder develops innumerable polyps in the colon, large areas of which come to resemble a carpet of tiny polyps of the adematous variety. These polyps may remain silent, bleed, or

TABLE 5.1 Calcium-rich Foods*

Item	Serving Size	Calcium (mg.)
Sardines, with bones	3 ounces	372
Skim milk	1 cup	296
Whole milk	1 cup	288
Yogurt	1 cup	272
Swiss cheese	1 ounce	262
Cheddar cheese	1 ounce	213
American cheese	1 ounce	198
Oysters	¾ cup	170
Salmon, canned with bones	3 ounces	167
Collard greens	½ cup	145
Cottage cheese, creamed	½ cup	116
Spinach, cooked	½ cup	106
Ice cream	½ cup	97
Mustard greens, cooked	½ cup	97
Corn muffin	2 medium	90
Cottage cheese, dry curd	½ cup	90
Kale, cooked	½ cup	74
Broccoli, cooked	½ cup	68
Orange	1 medium	54

Source: Based on data in Agriculture Handbooks Nos. 8 and 456.

*Other foods high in calcium include almonds, bok choy (spoon cabbage), dandelion greens, dried fruits (most), legumes, molasses (black strap), mustard greens, okra, rutabaga, and turnip greens.

become ulcerated, but sooner or later their malignant potential turns them all into cancers.

Although familial polyposis is not a common illness, those with any family history of colonic cancer or early death from intestinal malignancies, should ask their doctors to screen for it at the annual checkup.

These tiny polyps are easily felt by your doctor during a routine rectal examination, and are readily seen in a sigmoidoscopic examination, which should be part of every annual physical. Only rarely do the polyps fail to extend low enough to elude these routine methods of detection.

Although in the past a partial colectomy was recommended, all authorities now agree that the danger associated with these polyps is so great that as soon as the condition is diagnosed, the entire colon, including the anus, must be removed. A newer operation, in which the entire colon is removed, preserves the rectal muscles and strips the lining out of the anus and rectum. This allows for preservation of the normal act of defecation, and thus presents a reasonable and practical solution to the medical and the cosmetic problems posed by treatment of this disease.

Colonic Cancer

The future of improvement in our treatment of colonic cancer must focus on prevention, because the overall survival from cancer of this organ has not improved significantly in the last 25 years. Thus the emphasis on the search for hidden colonic bleeding and colonic polyps by the entire medical profession, and which is underlined by the space devoted to these areas in this chapter.

The enormity of the problem is clear from these facts: In 1985 there were 138,000 new cases and 60,000 related deaths were estimated. Colon and rectal cancer develops eventually in 6% of the American population, and 6 million Americans alive today will die of it, divided equally between the sexes.

In terms of prevention it is reasonable to follow a diet high in fiber and roughage to prevent constipation. It seems prudent also to reduce the animal fats of your diet, which means a reduction especially of red meat, although this has not been proven beyond a shadow of a doubt. It has been proposed that dietary fat enhances cholesterol and bile acid synthesis by the liver, leading to increased amounts of these sterols in the colon. Colonic bacteria have a major role in converting these compounds to secondary bile acids (deoxycholic and lithocolic acids), cholesterol metabolites, and other potentially toxic metabolic products. Low dietary fiber intake and low fecal bulk contribute to an increase in the concentration of sterol metabolites in the stool and prolong their contact with the colonic mucosa. Population studies demonstrate an increased excretion of these products in groups consuming high-fat–low-fiber Western diets, as compared with other groups, and higher fecal bile acid levels have been found in patients with colorectal cancer than in controls.

Symptoms of Colonic Cancer

From what you already know about the colon, you can easily see that some of the symptoms of cancer of the colon will be caused by interfering with the movement of stool through the colon. Diarrhea is extremely rare; increasing constipation from the growing mass in the interior of the colon blocking the act of defecation is the more general rule. This holds true for the left side and lower portions of the colon just before the anus. In the right side of the colon, especially in the cecum, where the contents of liquid and the diameter of the organ is quite wide, there is less blockage of movement of the contents until the growth of the cancer becomes quite large and protrudes a great deal.

When *pain* develops, it is due to the contractions of the colon trying to empty itself, pushing, so to speak, on a closed or closing door. Even before pain, a sense of pressure can be felt throughout the entire organ, reaching down into the rectum.

Often persons will experience the urge to pass small formed, not watery, stools frequently, resulting from the partial hold up of colonic contents as thcy movc toward the rectum.

However, pain may never be felt. This is especially true when the growth is in the cecum and the tumor remains silent. So this warning sign is missing.

Bleeding and *anemia* are important signals of a possible cancerous growth. Visible blood, which varies in color from port wine to bright red, calls for a full-scale search for the cause. Unfortunately, the tumor may often shed only microscopic amounts of blood, which may not be seen by the naked eye. This is especially true in lesions of the right side of the colon, in the cecum most frequently. In this case, the slow development of *anemia,* with its attendant general weakness and shortness of breath, may be the only clue to the presence of a tumor. You may even experience some discomfort in the chest from the anemia, and think that your heart is not working normally.

CHANGES IN BOWEL PATTERN

Although your pattern of having a bowel movement may change as the result of trivial causes, any persistent change from your usual habits, whatever it may be, deserves looking into. This may be the only clue to the presence of a cancer early on in the colon.

Since persons pay attention to the shape of their stools, it is important to remember that a flat or ribbonlike stool does not point toward cancer. It is most often the result of narrowing of the rectum and colon as the consequence of a spastic contracted irritable bowel. This is like the shape toothpaste takes as it is squeezed out of varying shaped tubes.

Diagnosis

Any one of these obvious symptoms, or just the discovery of hidden bleeding during the course of a routine physical examination in which a fragment of stool is removed from the rectum during the routine finger rectal examination, is good enough reason to have a prompt sigmoidoscopic examination of the lower left side of the bowel, following good cleansing of the colon. This should be followed by a barium enema examination of the remainder of the colon, no matter what is found or not found on the left side.

Some physicians comfortable with and skilled in the use of the flexible colonoscope may prefer to make the search for colon cancer with this instrument, as was the case with President Reagan's physicians.

Whatever the technique used, if any suspicious area is seen on the x-ray or colonoscope, a biopsy should be taken of the area. Since cancer develops from polyps, it may be necessary to take several biopsies of suspicious areas, since some may show only the benign polyp portions and not the true malignant cancerous part.

Prognosis of Cancer of the Colon

The chances of survival and cure of colon cancer depend on what stage it is discovered. These stages are classified according to a series of so-called Duke's stages. As we have all learned from our national press articles about President Reagan's cancer of the colon: A Duke's stage A tumor is one confined to the lining layers of the colon, Duke's B is one that has penetrated into the wall of the colon beyond the lining layer, and Duke's C is one that has pierced through the external wall of the colon and reached the local lymph nodes draining the colon.

If the person has a Duke A tumor, the chances are between 85–95% cure if the cancer is removed surgically; in Duke B, the chance of cure is between 60–65%; and Duke C is reduced to 40%. These figures hold for whatever area of the colon the cancer is in.

Treatment

The treatment of colon cancer is surgical removal of the tumor and the lymph nodes draining the area involved. There is no real alternative. Even if the tumor has spread beyond the colon, it is necessary and desirable to reserve it to treat the bleeding and mechanical blockage the cancer is causing.

Radiation doesn't help and may even cause serious damage to the adjacent bowel and the organs within the abdomen. *Chemotherapy* has not been shown to improve the cure rate when given along with surgery or after it has been done.

If the tumor has spread to distant organs, the liver being the one most frequently involved, and the outlook is quite grim, there is a place for chemotherapy to slow down the growth of the cancer, and radiation can give relief of pain in bones if the tumor is there.

In almost all stages, cancer of the colon itself can be removed in a one-stage operation, which does not require any temporary or permanent external opening of the bowel (colostomy).

Cancer of the rectum, because of its special location, requires separate discussion. Although it rarely causes pain, cancer of the rectum does interfere with bowel movements by blocking the interior of the organ. Bleeding is very common and should not be mistaken for bleeding hemorrhoids (even if you know you have them) unless you have been carefully examined just recently.

Cancers of the rectum do not require very sophisticated tools to be detected. A careful rectal examination by your doctor with his or her finger finds the overwhelming majority of them. Sometimes your doctor will have you squat and bear down during the examination to bring the lower rectum and sigmoid colon further down. Before treatment of a rectal tumor is carried out, it is imperative that the lesion felt by your doctor be biopsied; sometimes it must be biopsied more than once to be sure of its exact nature.

Treatment of cancer of the rectum consists of surgical removal of the rectum followed by a colostomy. Understandably, loss of your rectum can be difficult to accept, but it's the only way we now have to insure a cure of this cancer. To do the colostomy, the surgeon creates an opening, or "stoma," in the left side of the abdomen, where the end of the sigmoid colon empties its contents.

Some medical centers are trying to find out if x-ray treatments before surgical removal of the rectum will improve the result of present-day operative techniques, but the results are not yet in. The hope is that this combined form of treatment will result in less widespread destructive removal of tissue around the rectum. It is this extreme kind of removal that may lead to damage to pelvic nerves and sexual function, especially in men.

Some individuals may need to wear a plastic appliance over the "stoma," but often it requires no more than a gauze pad. These sigmoid colostomies are emptied out daily with an irrigating device similar to an enema bag, and often they establish an automatic pattern.

To spare the victim of rectal cancer, especially the elderly and the debilitated, from having to adjust to a colostomy, the doctor may fulgurate the tumor; that is, burn it out piecemeal by an electrical cauterization. This is not the treatment of choice, because it requires multiple attacks on the tumor and does not offer the prospect of cure. However, it is a useful way of palliating the condition. It should be used only rarely because the tumor can and does recur, and a few patients have lived long enough to require a colostomy after all.

6

Diverticula, Diverticulosis, and Diverticulitis

Pockets and Boils

Diverticula

The colon is composed of two groups of muscle layers: an inner, circular layer that surrounds the colon and an outer, longitudinal layer. Although they may occur anywhere along the gastrointestinal tract, diverticula (diverticulum, singular) are most often found in the colon. They are little pouches that line the outer layer of the colon and are formed by its inner and outer layers. They occur at weak points in the colon's wall. When pressure in the colon rises as the muscles contract to move the contents along, these thin-walled sacs balloon through the outer wall (Figures 6-1, 6-2). The location of the diverticula is not due to chance; they form where the blood vessels that supply nutrition and oxygen to the colon enter the bowel and pierce its walls, creating areas of potential weakness.

Diverticulosis

Anyone can develop diverticula, a condition known as *diverticulosis*. This term simply means the condition of having diver-

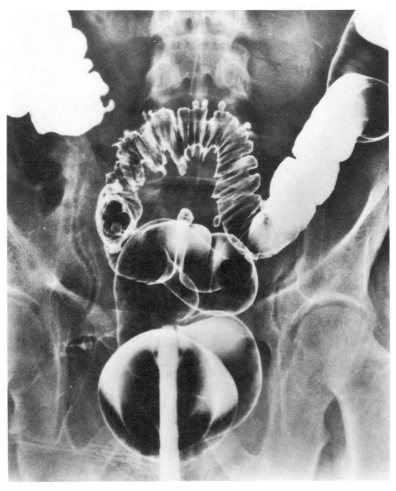

FIGURE 6.1 Barium enema showing diverticula, the grapelike outpouches.

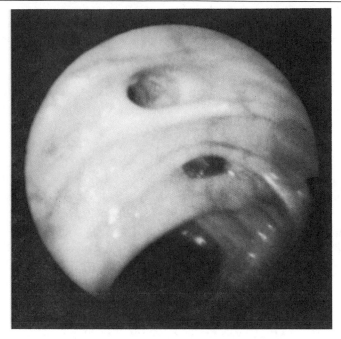

FIGURE 6.2 Diverticula of the sigmoid colon seen through a flexible sigmoidoscope. The dark circular and rectangular areas are the mouths of the diverticula. The scattered bright white dots are highlights of reflected light.

ticula and does not imply any inflammation or infection of them. Diverticulosis usually affects people in their forties and fifties, although it can occur in those both younger and older. It is hard to know how frequently it actually does occur. In Western nations, they may occur in as much as 10–15% of individuals studied by x-rays for any reasons. Once these pouches develop, they do not multiply or disappear and so remain a potential threat in that area.

Because these pockets need room to extend outside the muscle walls of the colon, they can occur only in the part of the colon that lies within the peritoneal cavity of the abdomen.

The colon can be thought of as a cylinder of varying widths, the cecal area being the widest and the sigmoid area the narrowest. Because the smaller a cylinder's diameter, the greater the pressure exerted on its walls, diverticula are most common in the sigmoid and least common in the cecum. They may also be scattered along the transverse colon, which has an intermediate width. This does not mean they cannot occur in the cecum, because they do on occasion, but only with great rarity.

Mainly through the work and clever thinking of one individual, D. P. Burkett, an English physician working in Africa, it has been realized in recent years that diverticulosis of the colon is much rarer in certain parts of the world than in others. Burkett found that diverticulosis is very rare in parts of the underdeveloped world, such as certain areas of Africa. He hypothesized that this might have some connection with the diet of the natives. The striking feature of these diets is their high fiber content.

If the diameter of the narrower segments of the colon is increased by the bulk of the diet, then the pressure on the wall of those segments will be lowered and the risk of developing diverticula decreased. Conversely, in low-bulk diets the diameter of the narrow segments of the colon remains unchanged and the possibility of developing diverticula increases.

Even before potential diverticula become actual ones, the wall of the colon in the sigmoid area reacts to the constant increased pressure. Like any other muscle in the body that is stretched by exercise, the colonic muscles respond by getting thicker. This *prediverticular phase* of thickened muscle wall with few diverticula can be seen on an x-ray and gives a characteristic "picket-fence" appearance (Figure 6.3).

To summarize, diverticula of the colon develop in areas of potential weakness where blood vessels pierce the walls as the result of the force exerted by the muscular layers. This force is lowest in the widest portion of the colon, the cecum (where the contents are mainly fluid) and highest in the narrowest area of the colon, the sigmoid (where the contents are more solid). Because of constant pressure, the muscle wall thickens in the narrow areas and balloons out the thin inner and outer layers of the colon, and gives rise to

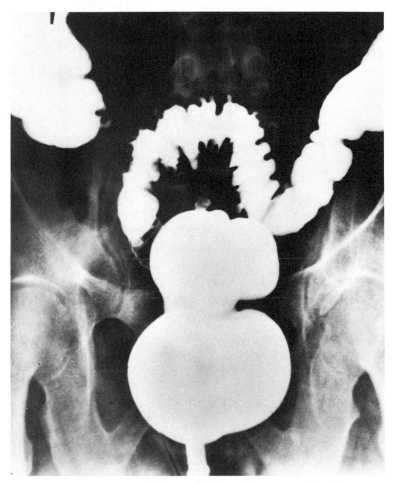

FIGURE 6.3 Barium enema of sigmoid colon, showing "picket fence" appearance of the thickened muscles of diverticular disease.

diverticula. It is believed that a diet high in fiber lowers the pressure on the colonic wall because it increases the width of the organ.

What Harm Can Diverticula Cause?

Although diverticula pose no problems to the great majority of individuals who have them, they may present problems for some.

The major complications of diverticula or diverticulosis are the *infection* in the pockets diverticulitis; the *perforation* of a pocket, and *bleeding* from the mouth of an individual diverticulum.

What Is Diverticulitis?

It is not having the irritable bowel syndrome plus the presence of a few diverticula in the sigmoid colon seen on an x-ray or by the sigmoidoscope. It is not having some distress in the left lower side of the abdomen with the muscle thickening of the *prediverticular* condition described in the preceding pages. It is a much more serious condition. *Diverticulitis* is an inflammation of the pockets of the diverticula with the development of an *abscess* (or boil) in the wall of the colon.

No one knows why or how quiet diverticula, which you may not even know you have, become inflamed, but it is thought that drv, hard stool gets caught in the pockets, interfering with blood supply and allowing the bacteria that are normally always there to infect the damaged tissue and form the abscess.

The symptoms of diverticulitis can vary a great deal in severity. Sometimes they may be mild with a slight abdominal discomfort that becomes worse when you are examined or press on the lower left side of your abdomen. You almost always will have a fever, which may only be low grade at first. The pain may become more intense and persist even if you are not being examined or even if you exert no pressure on that side of the abdomen. Sometimes the pain occurs on the right side of the abdomen, either because of diverticula in the cecum or because the sigmoid colon that has the diverticulitis is a floppy organ and may curl around to the right side of the peritoneum. In this case, you may wonder if you have appendicitis, and your doctor may be puzzled if you still have your appendix.

The swelling of the colon wall in the area of the diverticulitis can increase in size so that your doctor can feel it as a mass on physical examination; the area is very tender to the touch.

Diagnosis of Diverticulitis

The possibility of diverticulitis is raised by your story of abdominal pain, and its probability as being the cause is strengthened by the gentle examination of your abdomen by your doctor. Some *routine* laboratory studies help: a blood count to see if the white blood cells reflect an infection in your body and a plain x-ray (without any barium contrast material) to outline the colon, which often contains gas.

If a mass is felt or suspected, your doctor may order a sonogram, the sound wave examination like the sonors used under water, which does not use x-rays, to pinpoint his or her suspicion. Lately, CAT scans have become popular and are safe.

Too often a barium examination of the colon, the barium enema, is ordered before the diagnosis is clear. This type of examination, with its preliminary cleansing enemas and cathartics, is extremely dangerous and should be avoided. I feel that even the sigmoidoscope may be a dangerous instrument to pass into the inflamed colon.

Sometimes when the question of a perforation or partial perforation of the colon comes up, then a watery dye is slowly run into the rectum and x-rays taken to see if a leak in the colonic wall really exists.

Treatment

The immediate aim of treatment in the acute stage of diverticulitis, whether mild or severe, is to rest the bowel (reduce its work and contractions) and control the infection. To accomplish the first, your doctor will stop your regular solid food diet, replacing it with liquids only and to do the second, he or she will use antibiotics.

Except in the mildest cases or when your doctor is quite sure that you are having a very mild recurrence of your known diverticular disease of the past, most patients with diverticulitis need to be treated in a hospital in order that you may rest your bowel by receiving all your nourishment and fluid requirements by intravenous injections. The second reason for hospitalization is to give you the needed large doses of antibiotics directed against the bacteria that live in the lower bowel.

If this medical program is successful, you will begin to feel better, your temperature will come down to normal, and your pain will subside. Along with these signs of improvement, your bowels, which ordinarily slow down or even shut down completely, will begin to open up. This may take some time and you will need to be patient, because you can recover completely from an episode of acute diverticulitis with current medical treatment.

At other times, however, the infection does not seem to be controlled by these methods, and the inflammation may begin to spread. It may impinge on the urinary bladder and give you urinary symptoms such as burning, or pain, or frequency of urination. Or the swelling of the colon wall may grow larger on physical examination, or when you are studied by the sonogram or CAT scan.

At this point, the question of an operation will arise. The focus of infection must be removed. This means two things: (1) the abscess must be drained (like any boil, the pus must be evacuated), and (2) that part of the sigmoid colon in which it arose must be removed. But beyond these two things, the area of the colon from which a portion has been removed (*resected* is the technical surgical term) must be protected from the stool coming down from above, in order that the parts of the colon that were sewn together not become infected or put under mechanical stress or pressure. To do this requires that the intestinal contents be diverted to the outside of the abdomen temporarily by means of a colostomy (an opening in the colon to the exterior).

In most cases, this surgical treatment will require that the operation be done in two stages. At the first stage, the diverting colostomy will be performed and the resection of the sigmoid diverticulitis will be done. In the second stage, done several weeks later, the external opening to the abdomen will be closed and the bowel movements will again be passed through the rectum as usual.

In more urgent conditions, when it appears that the infection is spreading and peritonitis may be setting in, only the colostomy can be done in an emergency fashion. Thus two more operations may be needed: one to remove the sigmoid diverticula and the last to close the initial colostomy.

Nowadays with antibiotics, close medical attention, and good anesthesia, two-stage operations are all that are usually required.

Bleeding in Diverticulitis

The passage of bright red blood through the rectum is very unusual in acute diverticulitis, but it can occur from inflammation of the mouth of one of the diverticular pouches. The more usual situation is one in which you have rectal bleeding without pain, and a barium enema and/or sigmoidoscopy shows the presence of diverticula. Although this can occur, your doctor will take pains not to fall into the trap of stopping the search for other causes of rectal bleeding. You will have to accept the necessity for other and tedious examinations to be sure where the blood is coming from.

Perforation

The colon wall may become so inflamed that it develops a hole. This perforation may empty into the peritoneal cavity (a "free" perforation) or be walled off by the surrounding organs (a "contained" perforation). Both kinds of perforation urgently require an operation. Occasionally, the inflamed pocket of diverticulitis can actually penetrate into the adjacent urinary bladder, forming a hole into the bladder. This kind of connection is called a *fistula*. This perforation is quite painful and causes urinary tract infections. Treatment consists of an operation to close the hole in the bladder (it's rare that any part of the bladder will have to be removed), and the sigmoid diverticulitis from which the hole arose is removed. This may not require even a temporary colostomy.

Diverticula in Inflammatory Bowel Disease (IBD)

Since left-sided colonic diverticula are common and IBD occurs on the left side of the colon, it's not surprising that diverticula and IBD, such as ulcerative colitis and Crohn's disease, can coexist. The presence of diverticula in an individual with ulcerative colitis causes no difficulties, as ulcerative colitis is easily diagnosed by endoscopy.

The situation is different in Crohn's disease, however. Often it is difficult to decide whether the individual has severe diverticular disease with local extension (especially if the bladder is also in-flamed) or has Crohn's disease, and also happens to have a few diverticula. In these cases an operation may be required if the person is sick.

Prognosis

In most cases, the first attack of acute diverticulitis responds to bowel rest and antibiotics. Although no one can predict whether the disease will recur, it is a good preventive measure to go on a very high-fiber diet (30 grams/day) after the diverticulitis has cleared up.

People who have had a bad attack but have recovered with antibiotics are usually fearful of a recurrence, and with good reason. If their interval barium colon examination shows marked residual deformities, or if they have low-grade, persistent distress, they are better off having a one-stage operation, rather than risk a second severe attack, which may require a colostomy and one or two more stages of operation. These individuals, like those who have recovered from mild diverticulitis, should go on a very high-fiber diet.

Recurrences

Once you have had an acute attack of diverticulitis, you are sensitized to the possibility of a recurrence. Every pain in your lower left abdomen or disturbance in your bowel habits or feeling of lower abdominal tenderness could signal another major episode. What should you do if you suspect you are about to have a recurrence? This is an important question, especially when you are away from home and your regular doctor. If you have any of the symptoms described above, plus a fever: (1) reduce your food intake and drink only clear liquids, and (2) take antibiotics active against intestinal organisms, using one prescribed by your doctor and to which you are known not to react adversely. If your symptoms do not respond within 12–24 hours, you should consult your doctor. If you travel frequently, you should carry a thermometer so that you can monitor your symptoms and decide whether you need to consult a local doctor, and carry a supply of the antibiotics that worked in the past.

Cancer and Diverticula or Diverticular Disease

Diverticula do not predispose you to cancer of the colon or to precancerous polyps of any type, but they can cause two problems.

One is the difficulty of determining whether the rectal bleeding you may have is due to a small polyp or small cancer or to diverticula. A more important and more frequent problem is determining whether there is a small cancer in the sigmoid colon, when the latter is the seat of diverticulitis or is scarred as the result of previous diverticulitis. A person who has had typical episodes of diverticular disease for years may have yet another episode that lingers on. Especially among older people, who are at greater risk for colonic cancer, it's important to make sure the diverticulitis or its scars are not masking a tumor. Sometimes removing this segment of the bowel is the only way to determine whether or not cancer is present.

Sigmoid Resection for Diverticulitis: Long-term Results

A sigmoid resection is an effective way to prevent recurrence of diverticulitis. It ordinarily does not affect bowel control and the occasional looseness of stool it causes is all to the good. Since the resection may not remove all the diverticula in the colon, you may wonder if those left behind will cause trouble in the future. The answer, interestingly and reassuringly, is no. Removal of the narrow sigmoid area together with a high-fiber diet protect you against recurrences, provided that the sigmoid form of diverticulitis was the cause of your original colonic symptoms.

Cecal Diverticulitis

Diverticula on the right side of the colon are rare because of the fluid content in that area and because the wide, open cecum has a lower wall pressure. Yet the cecum can develop diverticula which, like the appendix (which also arises from the cecum), can become inflamed, develop an abscess, and even perforate. Symptoms of appendicitis may in fact be caused by cecal diverticulitis. Even if you have no history of diverticula, you and your doctor will want to keep this possibility in mind. Whenever this situation arises, you should be operated upon promptly. "When in doubt, take it out" is a good slogan to remember about the symptoms of appendicitis.

Silent Diverticula

You may be discovered to have diverticula in your colon accidently, in the course of having an x-ray of your intestinal tract for other reasons. These diverticula may have no meaning and pose no threat to your health. If you have them but have no discomfort or signs of inflammation, you do not need any medical therapy. However, it would be wise to review your bowel habits, use of laxatives, your history of minor colonic discomfort, and especially your intake of fiber.

The Irritable Bowel Syndrome (IBS) and Colonic Diverticula

You may have all or some of the symptoms of the IBS discussed at length in Chapter 2, and be discovered to have some sigmoid diverticula in the course of the x-ray studies your doctor thinks are necessary to establish the diagnosis and rule out other colonic diseases. How important are they and do they need special treatment?

Remember that diverticula are common in the general population and probably have little to do with the symptoms of the IBS. If you have a long history of constipation and of taking laxatives, switching to a high-fiber diet is the best approach. You will need to consult the tables included in this book, (chapter 4,) to calculate how much fiber you are eating at present and increase it substantially. At least 30 grams of fiber per day is a good goal, although some individuals need more. Remember that you may experience abdominal discomfort in going from a low- to a high-fiber diet. Many people panic or grow impatient with the tempo of improvement and are tempted to abandon the effort, but this is precisely the time to stay with the high-fiber intake. If discomfort persists, ask your doctor whether he or she can prescribe an antispasmodic pill. This sometimes helps. Taking psyllium plant seed preparations such as Metamucil can also help during this transition. In view of the widespread popularity of Metamucil among doctors and patients, you might wonder why it's not routinely recommended to all individuals who need to increase their intake of bulk. Although these substances are harmless, it's preferable to try to improve dietary habits first before turning to other means.

7

Food Allergies

Fact and/or Fancy

The intestinal symptoms that arise from food intolerances and those that arise from disorders of the intestinal tract often overlap. Their differences become blurred at times. It seems appropriate, therefore, to discuss this area now to provide the reader with some guidelines for sorting out the differences and seeking the appropriate medical help.

How often after a meal that has made us uncomfortable do we not say "I must be allergic to something I ate," whether our symptoms are those of belching and burping, heartburn, "indigestion" felt in the upper abdomen and chest or lower abdomen, or cramps followed by diarrhea?

We know that we are using the word "allergic" very loosely. Sometimes we express our gastrointestinal reaction by saying "I can't tolerate" this or that food or drink, yet on another day we consume it without any bad effects. So we conclude that perhaps we have a limited tolerance for a certain article in our diet: We know that hay fever sufferers don't always sneeze when pollens are

146

floating around because the pollen count must be high enough to produce discomfort.

Can we sort out these differences? In all this loose talk and thinking can we find some definite facts? Are there really food allergies or is this only an old wives' tale?

No one doubts that food allergies exist, but because controversy and possible quackery surround the whole subject, doctors approach it with great caution. The major problem is that it is difficult to prove that the symptoms blamed on food allergies are really caused by foods. Common symptoms include (1) gastrointestinal symptoms (nausea, vomiting, abdominal cramps, diarrhea); (2) distant symptoms [hives, swelling of lips and throat, (angioneurotic edema) and eczema]; (3) asthma and swelling of the nasal passages; and (4) migraine. With such a diverse list you can see why your doctor might feel defeated even before beginning an investigation of possible causes.

Another reason why food allergies are difficult to identify is that the diagnostic tests are hard to interpret and unreliable. For example, *skin tests* in which extracts of the suspected foodstuffs are either pricked or scratched into the skin are widely used and equally widely suspected because they are unreliable. Recently, a great deal of energy and money has been spent on detailed chemical analyses of hair and fingernails in an effort to relate these findings to presumed nutritive deficiencies arising from disturbed diets. Although some understanding of the body's nutritional status, especially protein balance, can be gained from hair analysis, most of these expensive tests shed no real light on the nutritional causes being studied. Another group of tests, radioallergosorbent tests (RASTs) and the measurement of immunoglobulins of the blood, especially immunoglobulin E (IgE), have a better scientific foundation but are expensive and often not confirmative. As a result, patients, physicians, and nutritionists resort to *elimination diets*. Either specific foods (e.g., milk) or classes of food (e.g., wheat or dairy products) are forbidden or a few simple foods allowed and new foodstuffs gradually added. The elimination diet approach is widely used but difficult to follow given the daily demands placed on the actively employed individual.

Finally, food allergies are tricky to diagnose because the different kinds of reactions to food need to be separated and better defined. Recently, clinical researchers have made a start in this direction in an attempt to upgrade the scientific bases of the classification of these reactions.

Terms

Food intolerance, the most widely used term, covers the whole gamut of adverse reactions to foods and includes the two main groups: *food idiosyncracy* and *food allergy.*

Food idiosyncracy refers to a specific reaction to a specific food substance, perhaps based on a specific defect in the body's enzyme system. Phenylketonuria, a disease in which the newborn infant cannot handle a specific amino acid and which is tested for routinely at birth, is such an example.

Food allergy refers to an adverse reaction to food that satisfies two criteria: (1) the participation of a component of the immune system (often quite difficult to prove), and (2) the recurrence of symptoms on two or more occasions when the suspected food is retested.

However, it is often very difficult to decide whether an allergic factor is present even if you react badly every time you eat a specific substance. This gray area can include drugs as well as food. Aspirin sensitivity is a good example. The fact that some individuals react to aspirin with asthma or eczema suggests that an allergy is present, yet the mechanics that cause the reaction have not been shown to be immunological.

Food intolerances that occur every time an individual eats or drinks a specific substance may be due to a direct *chemical toxic effect.* Rapid heart beating after tea, coffee, chocolate, or cocoa, may result directly from the caffeine, theobromine, and methylxanthine in these beverages. Many individuals, especially Jews and blacks, experience bloating, "gas," abdominal cramps, and even diarrhea after drinking milk or eating dairy products (e.g., cheese, ice cream, butter). Further, other individuals, as they grow older, may develop these reactions to milk, although they did not experience them earlier in life. A considerable part of this intolerance to milk is due to the presence in milk of the sugar *lactose* (composed of one molecule of glucose and one molecule of galactose), which is split and digested by the enzyme *lactase* present in the cells lining the intestinal tract. The lack or reduction in the amount of lactase leads to some of the unsplit lactose reaching the colon, where the intestinal bacteria feed on it and produce gasses and irritating acids. *Lactose intolerance* is now widely known by the general public. Those who need to drink milk can partially correct the lactase deficiency by adding a special enzyme preparation to the milk. LactAid is one such available remedy. The difficulties some people have with milk may be related to other substances it contains, especially proteins. Milk contains at least 20 proteins and these can cause true allergic reactions.

Other substances such as wine may induce reactions, because toxic materials are released when they are left to stand around after being opened. Foods that contain histamine, such as fermented cheeses and sausages, or which contain histamine-releasing tyramine, such as chocolate, cheeses, and canned fish, can also produce reactions that mimic allergic reactions. Another food intolerance most people have heard of is the *Chinese restaurant syndrome.* Characterized by gastric distress, warmth, flushing, headaches, and dizziness; it is presumed due to the monosodium glutamate (MSG) contained in Chinese dishes, and it appears within 30 minutes after being eaten.

As you can see, the list of foods suspected of causing allergic symptoms is long. In one group of 100 patients, the following foods were involved (the number after the food is the number of patients affected): milk (46), eggs (40), nuts/peanuts (22), fish/shellfish (22), wheat-flour (9), tea and coffee (8), chocolate (8), artificial colors (7), pork/bacon (7), and chicken, tomatoes, soft fruit, and cheese (6 each).

Products that contain mold spores may also be a problem, and this includes highly aged cheese, wine, yogurt, and yeast.

True Food Allergies

Experiencing symptoms such as swelling of the lips or tongue, a runny nose, hives, asthma, or eczema, within minutes of eating a certain food is clear evidence of an allergic reaction.

If your symptoms begin more than an hour after eating the suspected food, it is more difficult to prove that they are caused by an allergy. The first thing to do is to be certain that these symptoms recur every time you eat the suspected substance. In addition to the symptoms mentioned above, those that may appear more than an hour after a particular food is consumed include such gastrointestinal effects as vomiting, diarrhea, abdominal pain, bloating, and constipation. Rarely, intestinal bleeding may be caused by an allergic mechanism. To rule out an intestinal disorder that can cause the same symptoms, your doctor should first take a careful history, give you a complete physical examination, and request all the appropriate laboratory tests.

Wheat Intolerance—Sprue—Gluten Enteropathy

Wheat or substances that contain the wheat protein called gluten, such as wheat-containing flour, bread, cakes, stuffings, pasta, and so on, appear frequently on the list of substances people cannot tolerate. Gluten is present also in rye, oats, and barley.

One disease, sprue, or coeliac disease, is a form of intestinal malabsorption that is clearly due to the inability of the individual's intestinal lining cells to handle gluten. This leads to malabsorption, weight loss, loss of fat in the stools, and often diarrhea and bloating. A chronic skin condition, dermatitis herpetiformis, also known as Duhring's disease, may also be associated with sprue or spruelike changes in the small intestine. The striking point here is that removal of the gluten from the diet leads to prompt restoration of health and disappearance of symptoms. The diagnosis rests not only on the good effect of withdrawing gluten from the diet, but on the fact that biopsies of the small intestinal lining reveal marked abnormalities that return to normal as the individual's health improves. In a few cases, people with *sprue* or *gluten enteropathy,* as it is technically labeled, need to remove lactose from their diets as well. Very rarely, even removal of these two major offenders is not enough, and other substances such as chicken and/or eggs must be eliminated from the diet.

We still don't know whether the sensitivity to gluten in sprue is purely an allergic (immunologically mediated) reaction or is also in part a toxic reaction. Before the discovery in the 1960s of wheat's role in sprue, this disorder was treated with cortisone to suppress a presumed immunological inflammation in the intestinal wall.

Mild Wheat Intolerance

Unlike sprue, mild wheat intolerance does not inflame the cell lining of the intestine, but it does cause intestinal symptoms such as bloating, gas, distention, and even diarrhea. There is no laboratory test to prove this condition, only the reactions of the individual to repeated attempts to eat wheat or wheat-containing foodstuffs.

Although almost everything we eat that is digested by the intestinal secretions is completely absorbed by the body, some starch is not broken down by the appropriate enzymes, escapes absorption in the small bowel, and reaches the colon. The amount varies from individual to individual and depends on the kind of starch. For example, the carbohydrate of rice flour is absorbed completely, whereas some of the carbohydrate of all-purpose white wheat flour is not. This malabsorption in some individuals can be corrected by withdrawing gluten from the diet.

This curious phenomenon is thought to be caused by an interaction between starch and wheat protein, which interferes with the former's complete absorption and thus produces unpleasant gut sensations. Until we better understand this problem, however, it is important not to fall victim to the many untested remedies that have been proposed, such as eating certain substances with only certain other substances; you risk developing a lopsided diet.

Food Allergies in Diseases of the Bowel and Colon

When the cause of an intestinal disease is unknown, it is natural to try to incriminate the food people eat. For example, there is a long history of unsuccessful attempts to find a food that causes ulcerative colitis. Sensitivity to cow's milk or premature weaning from breast feeding plus the early introduction of formula feeding have long been suspected as being important. Although neither theory has been proven, some doctors and patients still cling to the idea that milk may be dangerous in this disease. If there is something to this concept, and there may be in cases of childhood ulcerative colitis, it is probably the 20 or more proteins in milk, not the milk sugar—*lactose*—that play a role.

Accurate surveys of what people ate before they became sick are very difficult to obtain, especially in disorders that take a long time to develop. Still, that has not prevented researchers from also speculating on the role of dietary habits in setting the stage for the development of Crohn's disease. For some time they have suspected that sweetened breakfast cereals contribute to the onset of the disease, although more recently the focus has shifted to the role of a high-sugar *and* low-fiber diet. At present, studies are being conducted, especially in Great Britain, to assess the treatment of patients with Crohn's disease with high-fiber/low-carbohydrate diets. My advice is given specifically in Chapter 3, but, in general, when an individual with Crohn's disease does not have diarrhea or mechanical obstruction of the intestine, I urge a diet with moderate fiber.

Another curious and interesting intestinal disease in which allergic reactions to food may be involved is *eosinophilic gastroenteritis*. In this disease, the stomach and intestinal lining cells become crowded by eosinophiles, the naturally-occurring blood cells that are involved in allergic reactions. In addition to producing uncomfortable intestinal symptoms, this disorder causes the lining cells of the bowel to become "leaky," with the result that important protein constituents of the blood seep into the intestine from which they are passed out in the stool and so are lost to the individual. The level of blood proteins falls and swellings of the body occur— "edema"—especially in the legs. People so affected may have an increased number of eosinophiles in their blood as well, but not always. Some get better when milk, eggs, wheat, soy protein, or steak are removed from their diets, but others may require medicines as well.

How to Diagnose a Food Allergy

The first step in deciding whether your intestinal symptoms are due to an intestinal disorder or a food intolerance is for your doctor to eliminate those intestinal disorders and diseases that can cause identical symptoms. If this has been done, and you or your family have a history of allergies (such as eczema, hives, allergic asthma, or runny noes, etc.) it's more likely that your intestinal symptom is caused by a food allergy.

As noted at the beginning of this chapter, it's difficult to make a clear-cut diagnosis of food allergy; skin tests, for example, are unreliable. Your medical history is, of course, terribly important, especially if you can recollect the specific circumstances of an "allergic" episode (a dramatic intestinal explosion following strawberries or shellfish will never be forgotten!). Memory is not always reliable, however, so we come back to the old stand by—*elimination diets.* Tedious, boring, and difficult as they are to carry out, especially by busy people on the move, elimination diets offer the best way to diagnose a food allergy. If you undertake such a trial by diet, you will need to follow it religiously, keep detailed notes, and not give up after a few days. I believe any elimination diet must be followed conscientiously for at least 2 weeks.

Although your doctor may have his or her own recommendations, I suggest eliminating one and only one of the most common offenders at a given time: milk, wheat, egg, spices, perhaps nuts. For milk, it is not enough to switch to skim milk. You must eliminate all milk and milk-containing products, such as cheese, ice cream, yogurt, and butter. For cheese, there is no substitute, although recently an ice cream substitute containing tofu has become available. Nondairy creamers can be substituted for some of milk's uses. Margarine is a good substitute for butter, but you will need to look at the label closely to see that the product you select does not contain any milk solids (in the United States, Fleischmann's margarine is one such.)

If the elimination of one of these commonest offenders does do the trick, your future course is clear: You must eliminate that entire class of food from your diet. Because some reactions depend on the dose of the offending food, you might be able to tolerate a small amount. You will have to determine this yourself by careful testing, however.

What if these simple elimination diets do not help? If a few conscientiously followed trials do not work, you must consider the possibility that you do not have a dietary problem, especially if a full diet doesn't make you feel any the worse. If you and your doctor are convinced that food plays a part in your distress, however, there are a few more tedious trials and trails that you may want to follow.

One option is to go on an *elemental diet,* the kind of diet the astronauts have tried. These are expensive, not very palatable, prepared diets that are chemically pure. Vivonex is one such commercially available elemental diet, Flexical another. Because they are quite unpalatable, most people are unwilling to stick to them, but they are worth considering.

A more acceptable, although still difficult, approach is the "core diet." For about 20 years I have recommended this very restricted, though simple, diet to those concerned that their troubles are dietary. Only four substances are allowed and it's a good idea to stock up enough of each to last for 2 weeks:

1. *Bottled mineral water.*
2. *One starch* (either rice or potato but not both). (instant rice or raw rice can be cooked with the mineral water.)
3. *One meat* (either boiled, broiled, or roast chicken, or broiled lamb chops, but not both).
4. *One canned fruit* (I suggest Bartlett pears).

It is extremely rare for anyone to be sensitive to these few substances. This diet should be followed for at least 2 or preferably for 4 weeks until your intestinal turmoil subsides; only then can one new food be added every other day, with egg, wheat, and milk as the last to be added. If a new addition produces a reaction, you "back up" to the previously tolerated level and start in again after a week of stabilization.

You can see how this can be tedious and rather cumbersome to carry out, but some well-motivated individuals have been able to pinpoint the offending food or foods with this approach. But I should warn you that allergies of this type are not common.

Antiallergy Drugs

In general, drugs are not helpful except to provide symptomatic relief. Antihistamines of the two general types (Benadryl and cimetidine) have not worked in my patients, and one would certainly not use any more powerful antiinflammatory drugs. One drug that has had a vogue for immunologically mediated food allergy (IgE) is sodium cromoglycate (Cromolyn), marketed abroad as Nalcrom, but my patients and I have been disappointed in its use. Although for a while the Letters to the Editor section of several good medical journals contained anecdotes of the effectiveness of this substance, submitted by doctors who were treating themselves, I wouldn't send you abroad to get this material. In the United States, it is available as capsules to be used as inhalant for asthma in children, but the dose is too small to be worth a try for attempting to treat food "allergies," and the patient might need to take five capsules four times daily. This capsule contains lactose as well.

8

The Aging Gut

In the United States, the 65 and over age group is the fastest growing sector of the population and currently numbers about 28 million. According to careful population projections, by the year 2050
one out of every eight of us will be 75 years or older. What effect
does the normal aging process have on our gastrointestinal tract?

Normal Aging of the Intestines

As we age, many of us lose weight despite a good appetite, a good
diet, and the absence of any obvious diseases of the intestine or
other parts of the body. Part of this is because the intestine does not
function as effectively as it did in earlier years, and we consequently
absorb less of our intestinal contents. The long list of substances
that the body may no longer absorb as well as it once did includes
vitamin B_1 and B_{12}, vitamin D, vitamin A and its precursor substance carotene, and folic acid, the vitamin needed to build red
blood cells and hemoglobin. Fats too may fail to be absorbed as

well as when we were younger, and there are hints that the sugars of a carbohydrate breakfast are less well absorbed as we age.

In view of the current intense interest in calcium—because of its role in preventing osteoporosis in menopausal women and its possible role in lowering high blood pressure and even in protecting against colonic cancer—you should know it does seem reasonably certain that calcium absorption declines with age. The reasons for this are complex and include the failure of intestinal cells to function optimally, and the problems of diminished vitamin D absorption. By contrast, iron seems to be absorbed reasonably well in the older age groups, as are most drugs.

The causes of these variations with age are not clearly known. The aging liver makes normal amounts of bile, and the aging pancreas in its protected interior of the body makes adequate amounts of the enzymes needed for fat and protein digestion, so they do not help explain the decreased efficiency of the aging gut. Rather it is reasonable to believe that the cells of the intestine which absorb digested materials either are sparser as we age or do not function as effectively as they did earlier in life. It seems unlikely that the blood flow to the intestine is at fault as some have claimed.

Changes in the colonic bacteria may interfere with intestinal absorption with aging. These organisms may migrate upstream into the small bowel, causing so-called bacteria overgrowth, share the host's diet, and impair normal absorption with resultant diarrhea. Sometimes this may be due to the low acidity of the older stomach (acid normally acts as an antiseptic sterilizing agent) or disturbances in the "housekeeping" waves of motion, which normally sweep through the small intestine but fail to sweep this bacterial overgrowth out of the aging upper bowel. Some older individuals who are malnourished and have diarrhea have bacterial overgrowth without any apparent cause. Antibiotics may help these people greatly.

Colonic Function as the Colon Ages

People often experience an increased difficulty in moving their bowels with age. A gradual decrease in the amount of stool passed

becomes apparent around age 65. Some of this may be due to loss
of teeth and the choice of a softer, less rough diet; diminished food
intake (because it is boring to eat alone after the death of a spouse);
and changes in the intestinal muscular activity of the very old; as
well as diminished general muscular activity. This constipation may
also be the result of neurological degeneration, or the cumulative
effect of years of taking laxatives that were effective before, as well
as the effects of parkinsonism or the drugs used to treat parkinsonism.

What Part Does Aging Play in Ordinary Ills
the Intestine is Prone to?

In general, the aging intestine is subject to all the disorders discussed in this volume, with some variations. The irritable bowel
syndrome (IBS), the commonest disorder of the intestinal tract
(Chapter 2), is also the commonest in the older age group. As in the
younger groups, the danger is that IBS may mask an organic cause,
such as benign, or more seriously, malignant tumors. The important point is that IBS does not come on suddenly late in life; there is
almost always a long history of it.

Inflammatory bowel disease (IBD) (Chapter 3) ulcerative colitis
and Crohn's disease are characteristically diseases of young people,
but from all parts of the world reports indicate that a second wave
of these diseases can and does occur after age 50. Older people who
develop IBD may have a more stormy course and are at greater risk
for surgical complications. Just what triggers off IBD in older people is far from clear. It was once thought that perhaps diseases of
the blood vessels played a part, but this does not seem to be the
case. One could surmise that susceptibility to these disorders is
increased by a failing of an aged immune system.

The incidence of cancer increases steadily with age; it is not
primarily a disease of the young. It has been calculated that the risk
of developing a cancer at age 61 is about 1% and increases to 2% at
age 81, with men more likely than women to be affected. There is
some decline in incidence in the nineties, but it is still high compared with the incidence of cancer among the middle-aged. The

statistics for cancer of the colon follow the same general trend, although there is no difference in this cancer between men and women. The risk for cancer of the rectum and colon begins to rise slightly at age 40, and then sharply at age 50, doubling with each decade and peaking at age 75–80.

Polyps of the colon and rectum are rare before 30. After age 30, incidence gradually increases so that by age 60–70, as many as 60% of the population may have one or more polyps. There does seem to be a slightly greater incidence among men.

The incidence of *diverticula of the colon* in the West increases steadily with age, so that half of all people 90 or older have them. In general, diverticular disease and diverticulitis (Chapter 6) occur more frequently over 50 than below that age.

What about *diarrhea* in the aging population? We must distinguish clearly between *diarrhea* (having too many loose stools day or night) and *fecal incontinence* (the inability to control one's bowel movements). In contrast to constipation, which does increase with age, there is no tendency for older people to have more diarrheal problems. There are two examples of diarrhea in the aging population that are often not recognized and deserve comment.

People who have had their gallbladders removed sometimes develop loose stools. This can occur even years after gallbladder removal. Although the cause is not well understood, it seems to be due to excessive amounts of bile in the colon—almost as if they were giving themselves a purge. The bile can be treated quite effectively by gels or resin (cholestyramine, Questran) that bind bile.

The other form of diarrhea may also be related to the invasion of the small intestine by the bacteria that normally live only in the colon. Running rampant in the upper bowel, they disrupt normal digestion, break down bile salts, share the host's meals, and release irritating fatty acids and gases. Antibiotics directed against these unwanted guests can provide dramatic relief.

Fecal Incontinence

Fecal incontinence, the inability to control one's bowel movements with consequent soiling and accidents, is a most distressing symptom, which is demoralizing in the extreme. It develops in the very old, but can occur in earlier life. It occurs when the rectal sphincter muscles (Figure 1.3) lose their tone or the ability of the anal area to feel the presence of stool, gas, or fluid in the rectum decreases. As we grow older, the tone of our rectal sphincters grows slacker, and when it is markedly deficient, we can become incontinent. Fecal incontinence seems to occur more often in aged women than men, and can also be a problem in women in their thirties and forties, perhaps because of birth traumas and injuries.

The causes of this condition are many and often difficult to determine. They may include direct damage to the sphincters as the result of surgery or other injuries; childbirth itself, or as the result of poorly done episiotomies, and diseases such as scleroderma (progressive systemic sclerosis) and late stage of diabetes. In the elderly, rectal and anal surgery for hemorrhoids, repair of sphincters, and fistulas add to the problem of the gradual loss of muscle tone.

In recent years we have made progress in treating this condition, which was once considered hopeless. Better medicines to slow down and control the movement of material through the intestine and colon are now available. Biofeedback techniques to "re-educate" the sphincter, developed mainly through the ingenuity of Dr. Marvin Schuster of the Johns Hopkins Medical School, also offer a new method of treatment.

To appreciate how this technique works, it helps to understand the normal functioning of the sphincter. The lower end of the colon is protected by two sets of valves, the internal sphincter, which is under the control of the autonomic nervous system (and therefore not under our voluntary control), and the external sphincter, which *is* under our control (Figure 1.3). Normally when a piece of stool or some gas reaches the rectum, the internal sphincter relaxes, but the external sphincter contracts so we can control defecation until we are ready. In people unable to control their bowel movements, the internal sphincter relaxes normally but the contraction of the external (voluntary) sphincter is weak or even absent, and control is lost.

In the biofeedback training program, the patient can see a screen that records these internal and external sphincters responses as waves on a graph. The patient is urged to contract the external sphincter. Surprisingly, a large percentage of people improve their fecal control by this kind of training program.

Bleeding from the Aging Bowel—Vascular Malfunctions

One of the most discouraging and upsetting conditions to experience as we grow older is to bleed from the intestine and yet have our doctors tell us that x-rays and other tests do not show where the blood is coming from. The bleeding may be very slow and hidden, with only our becoming anemic as the clue, confirmed by finding chemical evidence of blood in normal-looking stools. Or we may bleed more briskly with black or reddish blood in our bowel movements. It is disappointing to have a barium enema, upper gastrointestinal series, and small bowel x-rays with barium, and to have no cause revealed, or to have the frequently present diverticula detected but not to know whether the blood comes from them.

It is now known that a little less than half of the cases of this kind of bleeding in people over 65 comes from curious malfunctioning of tiny blood vessels in the lining wall of the intestine. These are tiny dilated blood vessels with abnormal connections between the small arteries and the very small veins in the gastrointestinal tract. They can be thought of as a very small varicose vein or a collection of them. Sometimes they occur on the surface of the skin or under the tongue, but most often they give no external clue. They have many names, but at present *angiodysplasia* is the most widely used one. This term simply means that the parts connecting the arteries to the veins are assembled incorrectly.

This condition can be detected by endoscopic examinations of the intestinal tract, especially by colonoscopy, since the right side of the colon is where the majority of these lesions are located in people over 60 years of age. Indeed it has been estimated that at least a quarter of individuals in this age group have these malformed blood vessels, but most do not bleed from them.

They can often be seen by the endoscope, but not always. It helps the physician find them if they are bleeding or have a clot over them, but this is not often the case. A scanning test with the subject's own red cells can be helpful. An x-ray of the blood vessels with dye (an angiogram) should rarely be done unless the scan is positive, because of the risks and a high failure rate if the scan is negative.

If the bleeding is serious, part of the colon, most frequently the cecum and right side, is removed. If the situation is not so urgent, your doctor will cauterize and coagulate these lesions by electric cauterization or laser beam techniques. The problem with all of these vascular lesions of the colon is that there may also be lesions in the stomach and small intestine. As a result, removal of the colon may only temporarily or partially solve the problem.

Some angiodysplastic blood vessels are probably congenital, whereas others occur in people who have associated defects in their blood clotting systems. Some people with angiodysplasia have other disorders of the circulation, especially lesions of aortic valves of the heart; these, too, suggest a hereditary cause. Despite the increased number in the older age groups, all people do not bleed. This may be related to the increased fragility of our blood vessels as we grow older. Since we can do little about this aspect of aging, the best strategy is for people to lower the pressure in their colon by the high-fiber diet advocated in Chapters 2 and 6 for the irritable bowel syndrome and diverticular disorders of the colon.

The Aging Blood Vessels of the Intestine and Colon

We all know that the chances of developing heart disease increase with age, mainly due to atherosclerosis, or hardening of the arteries of the heart. The other factors that increase our risk of developing heart disease have also been widely publicized: high blood pressure, diabetes, obesity, cigarette smoking, elevated blood cholesterol and fats, and the general effect of our genetic inheritance. When the circulation of blood to the heart muscles cannot keep up with their need for oxygen and nutrients, we can develop pain in our chest. This pain, *angina pectoris,* which simply means pain in the chest, comes on with effort (running after a bus, walking up stairs, or walking into a wind) or even, at times, at rest.

In a similar fashion, we can feel abdominal pain when the blood supply to the intestines does not keep up with their needs. This pain is similar to angina pectoris and is called *abdominal angina.* Advanced age (70+ years), high blood pressure, diabetes, and cigarette smoking, predispose a person to this condition, which seems to occur more frequently in women than men. The pain arises when the flow of blood to the intestines when they need it most (mainly while digesting a meal) is inadequate.

This discomfort is hard to diagnose by physical examination and the usual x-ray and endoscopic tests we have at our disposal, so the history you give your physician and your own observations are most important. In the course of digestion, *abdominal angina* is felt in the upper abdomen and around the belly button, coming on 15 minutes to 1 hour after a meal and subsiding after 1 to 4 hours. You try to get comfortable by changing your position or attempting to move your bowels or taking home remedies such as antiacids, but they do not help.

The more you eat the more it hurts, so you learn to cut down your food intake and thus lose weight. Occasionally you may have diarrhea as well. The net effect is that you begin to worry that you have a cancer in your abdomen. Because the ordinary x-ray and test do not help here, your physician begins to suspect that you do have a cancer, perhaps of the pancreas. But again the modern sophisticated tests: CT scans, ultrasound studies, endoscopy of the pancreatic duct turn up no clues. So you can appreciate how important is your close observation of the timing of pain and the act of eating.

The only way to make the diagnosis conclusively in this situation is to demonstrate that there is hardening of the arteries that supply the intestine, due to narrowing near the mouths of these vessels, which arise from the aorta, the main abdominal feeding blood vessels. This can only be done by an *angiogram,* an x-ray taken while a dye is injected into the intestinal arteries by a catheter inserted through a large vessel in the groin. This is not a pleasant experience, but the real risks are those of bleeding at the site where the artery was punctured for the test and, more serious, the risk of forming a clot, a thrombosis in the blood vessel, or pushing such a clot or a fragment of it into the circulation. You can see why this test is not lightly or frequently advised when abdominal angina due to hardening of the intestinal arteries is suspected, especially for older individuals who may have poor circulation to the heart and brain.

If the diagnosis can be proven, however, then a variety of surgical reconstructions or bypass operations can be done with improvement in the sufferers' pain and general debility.

Other Vascular Diseases of the Colon (Ischemic Colitis)

Another disturbance of the colon associated with aging is a form of colitis caused by vascular aging. Changes in the blood vessels result in diminished blood flow to the colon, whose tissues become damaged and inflamed. *Ischemia* is the word used to describe inadequate blood supply to an organ, and this form of colitis is thus called *ischemic colitis*. Often it is confused with the nonspecific forms of IBD (discussed at great length in Chapter 3). Ischemic colitis usually affects both men and women equally at about age 70, but is increasingly seen in individuals over the age of 50. Recently we have also learned that it can occur in young women in the small intestine and the colon. In these cases it seems to be associated with the use of the contraceptive pill. In older individuals, ischemic colitis appears in those whose hearts are simply not pumping enough blood to the intestine or who dislodge a clot from the heart to the intestine or form a clot in an intestinal blood vessel.

This condition is marked by the sudden onset of abdominal pain, nausea and vomiting and, most typically, bloody diarrhea. It can be diagnosed by x-ray study with barium or by endoscopy. The areas involved usually go on to complete healing, but occasionally they heal with a scar that causes a stricture of the bowel and may require a local operation to remove the narrow, scarred area.

9

Intestinal Repercussions of Other Diseases

General Diseases with Intestinal Repercussions

You must not assume that because your intestine is upset, the cause must be solely in the intestine itself. The intestine often responds to disturbances from other areas of the body. It is these intestinal repercussions I want to discuss now.

The *endocrine glands,* which secrete chemical messengers that reach all the cells of the body, may be lurking in the background of some of your discomfort. If one doesn't look for them, one will never discover them. The *thyroid gland,* which influences the metabolism of the entire body, can push the intestine too fast or slow it down too much. In *hyperthyroidism,* the overactive gland that we all recognize in the patient with staring "pop-eyes" can speed up the intestine and make the patient have too many and often too loose stools as material moves at breakneck speed through the intestine. But this disorder may be present in more subtle forms, the so-called *masked hyperthyroidism.* The older person does not look like the overactive, hypermanic individual and may even be apathetic. However, simple blood studies can easily help to ferret them out. On the other hand, the underactive thyroid with resultant *hypothyroidism* can cause weight gain, sluggishness, coarse skin, and poor hair growth. Constipation may be an important prominent result, with the other symptoms not at all apparent. Here again, simple, easily available blood studies will settle the question. In both instances the appropriate treatment of the overactive and the underactive thyroid gland will regularize and restore to normal function the disturbed bowel.

Diabetes, the disturbance in sugar and carbohydrate metabolism which, in those who develop it in adult life, is due to deficient insulin secretion from the pancreas, can after many years interfere with the normal functioning of the intestine. This happens because of the degeneration of nerves to the gut and disturbance in its ability to contract and move its contents along, loss of sensation from the rectum and anus, and loss of control of the rectal muscles. So loss of control and diarrhea can develop as well. These individuals may, unfortunately, also have problems with the emptying of their urinary bladders. The *diarrhea* is due to a number of factors, including nerve damage and the overgrowth of the intestine by intestinal bacteria. The *incontinence* is related as well to weakness of the anal sphincter muscles. However, broad spectrum antibiotics, binding of bile by resins such as cholestyramine (Questran) and the use of diphenoxylate (Lomotil) or loperamide (Imodium) often help control this problem, especially the troublesome nighttime diarrhea.

On the other hand, persons with diabetes with nerve involvement often complain of *constipation,* which is believed due to the disturbed autonomic nerve control of the intestine. This condition may also respond to treatment with newer medications, which act directly on the smooth muscle of the colon.

The *parathyroid* glands, four tiny glands near or embedded in the thyroid on the neck, play a central role in regulation of calcium metabolism and the blood levels of this important substance. When the blood level of calcium is elevated above normal with an overac-

tive parathyroid gland, constipation and abdominal pain may occur. Sometimes the severe abdominal pain due to overactive parathyroid gland and elevated blood levels of calcium can be due to
acute pancreatitis. Treating the parathyroid glands will arrest or
prevent the intestinal complications.

Finding out whether these general disturbances are having
repercussions in the intestine is easier nowadays with the routine
use of blood screening tests and the automated technology of medical laboratories. Disorders of these endocrine glands that we have
been discussing are turning up frequently because of the routine use
of automated comprehensive blood tests, even before they are suspected clinically. Often the isolated finding of an elevated or abnor-
mally low value may not have grave significance, but in the presence of intestinal symptoms your physician will make the effort to
determine whether these findings have any real meaning. They may
lead to a prompt solution for your intestinal dysfunction.

More Obscure Abdominal Disturbances, More Obscure Diseases

One can have recurrent attacks of severe abdominal pain, which
even our high-powered modern diagnostic tools are at a loss to
explain. *Acute intermittent porphyria,* in which the individual is
perfectly normal between attacks, is one such obscure disorder, but
has excruciating abdominal pain that comes on with lightning
rapidity. The passage of urine, which turns a dark red on standing,
may point to the diagnosis, which will be confirmed by blood and
urine tests. Doctors also look to the nervous system for possible
neurological causes of abdominal pain. Two that are usually
brought up are *abdominal migraine* and *abdominal epilepsy,* and
both are difficult to diagnose with certainty. These terms express
the idea that the sufferer is experiencing in the abdomen the equivalent of what he or she might have ordinarily experienced in the
head or nervous system, that they are having the equivalent of
migraine or epilepsy.

In *abdominal migraine,* periods of yawning, listlessness, or
drowsiness precede the abdominal attack. There may or may not be

a history of migraines or headaches in the individual, although there is most frequently a family history. The sufferer of abdominal migraine may have only the smallest headache, which is over-shadowed by the abdominal pain that lasts often for many hours and may recur in a row of attacks. There is no specific laboratory test for this disease, but an electroencephalogram during an attack or shortly after may show abnormal brain waves. The diagnosis is confirmed if the sufferer responds to the drug therapy of migraine.

Abdominal Epilepsy

Some episodes of electrical seizures of the brain are associated with abdominal complaints, and so the idea has arisen that some attacks of abdominal pain may represent an equivalent to a convulsion or electrical discharge from the brain. In the absence of a real mus-cular seizure, it is difficult to make this diagnosis. In some indi-viduals, however, attacks of pain with no evidence of organic dis-ease and with ever transient disturbance in feeling states or con-sciousness ("blackouts" that are fleeting), one could look into this possibility. An electroencephalogram here too will help if charac-teristic recordings are reported. This may require more than one study and, in the end, a trial of anticonvulsive medications may be attempted.

10

Medicines and the Gut

Diet, Drugs, and Disease Affect the Absorption of Medicines

Remember that every pill we take by mouth must pass out of the stomach and enter the small intestine for it to be absorbed into the system. Some drugs need to reach the colon to exert their effect. These include the antiinflammatory drug salazopyrine and its active component 5 aminosalicylic acid.

In addition, the presence of food in the intestine or the drugs themselves may affect the absorption of other medicines. Some antibiotics are less well-absorbed in the presence of food and should be taken either an hour before or three or more hours after a meal. These include penicillin, erythromycin, lincosyn, isoniazid, and tetracyclines (Table 10.1).

Some ions in food, mainly calcium (in milk and dairy products) and iron (in iron-enriched cereals and red meat) bind tetracyclines and therefore should not be taken within 2 hours of these foods.

Two drugs can specifically impair the absorption of the vitamin

TABLE 10.1 Influence of Food on Drug Absorption

Food Impairs Absorption of:	Food Enhances Absorption of:
Many antibiotics	Propanolol
Aspirin	Hydralazine
Propatheline	Hydrochlorothiazide
L-dopa	Propoxyphene
Methyldopa	Griseofulvin
Rifampin	Nitrofurantoin
Isoniazid	Spironolactone
Phenobarbital	
Methotrexate	
Acetaminophen	
Digoxin	
Furosemide	
Potassium ions	

folic acid, which is needed in the manufacture of the red iron cells and their hemoglobin. They are the anticonvulsant *phenytoin* (Dilantin) and the antiinflammatory salazopyrine. A long list of other drugs can interfere to limited extent with the absorption of other drugs (Table 10.2).

There is no problem in visualizing how *disease* of the gastrointestinal tract can interfere with the absorption of medicines and block their needed effects. Diseases of the pancreas and liver will affect the absorption of medicines that are absorbed along with fat; these are mainly the fat-soluble vitamins (A and D). Diseases of the small intestine, such as glutenenteropathy (sprue), or Crohn's disease can obviously prevent these vital substances taken from being absorbed.

In addition to disease, removal of a part of the small intestine can interfere markedly with the entry of drugs into the system. The clearest example is the removal of the terminal portion of the ileum for Crohn's disease (see Chapter 3). This is the place where vitamin B_{12} is absorbed from our diet. Although the normal liver usually contains enough vitamin B_{12} to keep up the supply for a few years,

TABLE 10.2 Drugs that Can Influence Drug, Vitamin, and Nutrient Absorption

Drug or Type	*May Affect Absorption of*
Antacids	Tetracycline
Antacids containing aluminum or magnesium in regular doses	Diazepan
	Cimetidine
Antacids in large doses	Nitrofurantoin
	Penicillin G
	Sulfa drugs
	Isoniazid
	Digoxin
	Phenytoin
	Chlorpromazine
	Propanolol
Antibiotics	
Tetracycline	Iron
Sulfasalazine	Folic acid
Antimetabolites	
Colchicine	Folic acid
	Vitamin B_{12}
Anticonvulsants	
Phenytoin	Folic acid
Oral contraceptives	Folic acid
Cholestyramine	Aspirin, chlorothiazide
	Iron, phenobarbital

disease and/or resection of ileal disease will take their toll, and the body's stores of vitamin B_{12} needs to be replenished periodically.

Drugs and Intestinal Function

In trying to understand new and unpleasant sensations in your intestine or definite clear-cut changes in bowel function, especially those that have come on recently, it is important to take an inventory of the medicine you are taking as well as changes in your dietary habits. We automatically think about new foods we have eaten, yet often forget to consider the effect of medicines we are taking, because we have been taking them automatically for so long a time that we never consider them. Remember that drugs can have cumulative effects as well as varied effects. It often takes some time and detective work to track this down.

Let us look at some of the commonly used medicines. A great many medicines we take for stomach distress for *upper* intestinal and abdominal discomfort, may react on and in our *lower* bowel.

Bismuth is one such substance very commonly taken in the form of Pepto-Bismol for gastric hyperacidity, nowadays having a marked revival for the treatment of traveler's diarrhea. This promptly causes the stools to become black, and may lead us to think we are bleeding from the stomach or duodenum.

If we are given iron pills because we are anemic due to blood loss, this too will cause our stools to become black and further confuse us as to whether we are still bleeding. In this instance, however, we have usually been warned by our doctors to watch out for this phenomenon. It is when we do not realize that we are taking iron in some mixture that we may become alarmed at the changes in the color of the stool. The commonest instance of this I see is the presence of iron in high-potency vitamin mixtures that also contain minerals, among them iron. Not so incidentally, we all ought to remember that some iron preparations can be very irritating to the bowels, causing cramps, or, more frequently, starting up constipation. Subjects with the irritable bowel syndrome and especially those with inflammatory bowel disease of any sort are prone to intolerance for iron-containing preparations. A variety of forms of iron are available and one may have to try several before finding one that is more easily taken. On rare occasions, iron may have to be given by intramuscular injections because of such marked intestinal intolerances.

As a result of the current emphasis on the need for adequate *calcium* in our diet, especially for menopausal women to avoid osteoporosis, lots of people are taking lots of calcium pills, and many may have some bad reactions. Again, cramps and constipation are the chief untoward effects. *Calcium carbonate* is widely recommended to prevent osteoporosis, and Tums is an inexpensive way of taking calcium carbonate. Occasionally, one will have to try out several forms of calcium pills before finding one that does not upset the usual bowel pattern. Remember also that if you are avoiding milk and milk products because of *lactose intolerance,* it does not make sense to take calcium in the form of calcium lactate, as may happen if you don't look carefully at the labels and package inserts of the calcium preparation you are currently using.

Tons of *antiacids* are bought and consumed daily in the United States for acid indigestion. Most of them have the same chemical lowering action in neutralizing the acid contents of the stomach. Their price, taste, and effect on the bowels vary. Those that contain *calcium carbonate* or the gel, *aluminum hydroxide* (Amphojel is one example of this latter group) usually quickly result in constipation. On the other hand, those that contain milk of magnesia (Maalox is one such) cause diarrhea.

All pain medicine that contains natural or synthetic forms of opiates, such as codeine or cough mixture that contains codeine, given for specific nonintestinal pain, cause constipation and bind up the bowels.

The newer acid-suppressing drugs like *cimetidine* (Tagamct or ranitidine (Zantac), widely prescribed for peptic ulcers of the stomach or duodenum, or more generously and loosely prescribed for any form of upper abdominal distress or "acidity," can cause looseness of the bowels and even more severe diarrhea.

Antidepressants are widely prescribed in our society. The group known as tricyclics are especially popular and can cause very marked constipation. One of the most likely offenders is the drug amitriptyline (Elavil), but the other antidepressants have similar effects, as well as interfering with emptying of the bladder, blurring of vision, and drying of the mouth.

The sugar *sorbitol,* which has a sweet taste but is not absorbed and thus is used in low-caloric hard candies, can be difficult to trace as the cause of loose stools. Here, keeping a list of everything we put in our mouths for a few days may give us the essential clue.

This book does not touch on disorders of the pancreas, but the abdominal pain and disturbances in the bowels that can occur in some forms of pancreatitis can be confused with other bowel feelings. *Diuretic pills* of the chlorothiazide type (Diuril is an example), which are frequently advised for women with premenstrual tension and weight gain because they cause the kidney to excrete more water and thus prevent retention of fluid, can be extremely difficult to track down as the cause of pancreatitis. This happens because they don't always cause pain every time they are taken, and they are not taken every day of the month, only in some prescribed premenstrual period.

Diuretics, "water pills" as they are commonly called, can also cause diarrhea, which may be very profuse and watery. This brings up a very sensitive subject, that of people who surreptitiously take diuretics in order to have diarrhea. Individuals who are driven by their need to lose weight in our fashion-conscious era, may also take laxatives as well. The sad part of this story is that they conceal these habits from those closest to them. Cascara and laxatives containing phenophothalein (Ex-Lax is an example) are the ones most commonly used. The other unfortunate part of the story is that until this is discovered, the individual will understandably be subjected to many expensive, tiring, and invasive tests. Some may even accept and undergo unnecessary operations in the vain search by their physicians for tumors of the pancreas, which may secrete substances that cause diarrhea.

An important group of medicines that can lead to intestinal and colonic inflammation, enterocolitis, are the *antibiotics*. There is no antibiotic, not even penicillin, considered one of the safest, or even erythromycin, which may not cause these disturbances, although the wide-spectrum antibiotics are the most feared and the most likely to upset the gut. They can start up as their mildest effect, simple diarrhea, labeled *antibiotic associated diarrhea,* and at their most damaging cause abdominal pain, diarrhea, rectal bleeding, and ulceration of the lining layer. These effects are the result of alteration in the kinds of bacteria and other organisms living in the colon. The ordinary inhabitants are suppressed and these "outsiders" proliferate. One group, the *Claustridia,* secrete a toxin that damages the mucosa and can form a coagulated cover on its surface, the so-called *pseudomembranous colitis.*

The problem with diagnosing these forms of colitis is that the antibiotic you have taken may have been forgotten, because the effects can take place even months later, and you need not have taken more than a few tablets to trigger this distressing sequence of events. Fortunately, the mild antibiotic-associated diarrhea will clear up by itself once the drug is stopped, and the more severe forms respond to measures that either bind the toxin (the resin cholestyramine [Questran]), or antibiotics such as metronidazole or vanconmycin hydrochloride (which destroys the *Claustridia*). Some chemicals used for the chemotherapy of cancer also can damage the colon, but this condition is easily recognized.

In the section on vascular disease of the gut, I have pointed out that in some few individuals the *contraceptive pill,* especially those that contain larger amounts of estrogen, induce clotting of the blood in the blood vessels supplying the intestine, and cause sudden abdominal pains, fever, and bloody diarrhea, so-called *ischemic colitis.*

Everyone knows by now that *aspirin* can cause an inflammation or ulceration of the stomach and duodenum, but aspirin can cause bleeding from even trivial lesions of the lower bowel because it interferes with the blood clotting system. One need not take very much aspirin for this to occur. Large numbers of men are now taking one aspirin tablet nightly to see whether it will prevent clotting of the blood in the coronary arteries of their hearts.

This kind of bleeding is even more likely when patients take anticoagulants, such as Coumadin, to prevent clotting or extension of a clot within the phlebitis of a leg vein, or after a clot has been thrown to the lung (*pulmonary embolus*) from the heart. It is not enough to stop the anticoagulant; one must make a search to find the lesion in the intestine from which the subject bled.

Intestinal Side Effects of Heart Treatment Medicines

Heart disease itself, especially the failing heart, can cause a great meny disturbances in the working of the bowel: constipation, sometimes diarrhea, and especially loss of appetite and thus weight loss and wasting. So it may be hard to separate the effects of the heart trouble from those caused by the medicines used to treat the heart disease.

Quinidine, used for disturbances in the heart rate, *Inderal* (the beta blocker propranolol) so widely used today for high blood pressure, angina pectoris, and disturbances in heart rate and rhythm, the newer calcium-channel blockers such as Procardia and verapamil (Colan) can all induce nausea, vomiting, diarrhea and most often constipation. The *diuretics,* "water pills," which can produce diarrhea and which are so important a part of the treatment of heart failure, should also be remembered in this connection.

Drugs and Porphyria: A Strange Cause of Attacks of Abdominal Pain

There is a strange, baffling, and obscure disease called acute intermittent *porphyria* based on a metabolic disturbance in the subject's liver, which needs to be considered in the cases of recurrent severe attacks of abdominal pain with distention and constipation. The pain can be terribly intense, suggesting an intra-abdominal catastrophe when none actually is taking place. The reason for considering it here is that attacks can be brought on by some very commonly used drugs: *barbiturates,* or *alcohol,* or *sulfa drugs.* The sudden onset, the severe pain, and associated nervous system symptoms of muscular weakness in the legs are frightening both to the sufferer and onlookers, especially because the commonly used diagnostic tests give no answers.

11

Intestinal Gas

What Is It?
Where Does It Come From?
What Can We Do About It?

We all seem to know what it is. We complain of belching and burping; we feel bloated and distended; we are embarrassed by passing gas through the rectum. There is an old, four-letter Anglo-Saxon word for this; more politely, we pass or break "wind." Our doctors use the more neutral word "flatulence" to describe this condition.

So what is the problem? Every temporary abdominal discomfort or unpleasant sensation we have is ascribed to "gas," whether or not accompanied by belching or flatulence. It is only relatively recently that we have come to know something substantial about intestinal gas, mainly through the work of one ingenious medical investigator, Dr. Michael Levitt, who devised methods for collecting, measuring, and analyzing the components of the gas present in the intestine.

Some things about gas we knew in the past. If we ate and talked, especially if we swallowed rapidly or gulped our food, we accumulated air in the upper stomach. If we sucked on a pipe or kept a cigar in our mouths for long periods of time or took deep "drags" of cigarettes, air could get trapped in the gullet or stomach. If we were constipated, we could understand how intestinal gas could pile up in the lower bowel. Certain foods were notoriously "gassy"—beans and members of the cabbage family especially. But this was about all a century of observation could tell us. Now we know a bit more. The gas within the intestinal tract is derived from three principal sources.

One is clearly room air, the atmosphere we all breathe. Mostly nitrogen, it contains the life-sustaining gas, oxygen. By being swallowed along with anything else we swallow, room air enters the gastrointestinal tract, but as it moves along the gut the amounts of nitrogen and oxygen change, as oxygen may dissolve in the blood and nitrogen may be added from the blood. The *second gas* in the intestine is carbon dioxide (CO_2), which is formed in the duodenum (the first portion of the small intestine [see Figure 1.1]) by a chemical reaction of the acid of the stomach (HCl) with the bicarbonate (HCO_3) of the pancreatic fluid. Soda bicarbonate in the stomach also can release carbon dioxide. Although the room air's nitrogen and oxygen and the carbon dioxide are odorless, the third kind of gas is not.

That *third source* is the lower bowel, the colon. Here the process of fermentation causes the formation of malodorous gases by the action of the normal colonic inhabitants, the local bacteria, on the undigested portions of our diet that have escaped absorption in the small bowel. These are principally carbohydrates, sugars, and some fat. From these are released such foul gases as methane or hydrogen sulphide (which has the odor of rotten eggs). In addition to the gases that arise from carbohydrates, Dr. Levitt has shown that there are interactions between unabsorbed starch and wheat flour, which also increase the amounts of gases found in the bowel.

From this account it is obvious that we can do certain things to help reduce the amount of gas we complain about. Some of us cannot talk volubly while dining. Most people eat too rapidly, gulping down air along with food. Smoking and chewing on a pipe stem or cigar must go. Many sufferers from belching and burping do not realize how much air they are swallowing, and need to change their eating habits. For others, anything that reduces the acidity of the stomach will help a bit in reducing the amount of carbon dioxide formed from the stomach's hydrochloric acid. So perhaps a blander diet and more nonabsorbable antacids (which do not contain bicarbonate and so do not release CO_2) will also be useful. The obvious gas-forming vegetables (beans, etc.) should be eliminated or their amounts reduced. For those who suffer a great deal from flatulence (and this can be more than a bad joke), drastic reduction in sugars in the diet and some reduction in starch (from potatoes and rice) and wheat flour (bread, cakes, and some pasta) are in order. Theoretically, reducing the colonic bacteria by intestinal antibiotics should work, but the risk of important side effects of these antibiotics in the gut and elsewhere make this method a theoretical approach and much too risky.

One of the most interesting and important facts discovered regarding intestinal gas is that the patients who complain continually of gaseousness are usually those who suffer from the severe forms of the irritable bowel syndrome (IBS) (discussed in Chapter 2). They feel that they make or have too much gas, but actually they do not. When these individuals are investigated by modern techniques, they have been shown to have just as much or as little gas as normal individuals. They are not making excessively large amounts of gas; it is just that they cannot tolerate these normal amounts of gas in their intestine. Their threshold for sensitivity to distention is lower than the average nonsuffering individual. The same amount of gas gives them pain and discomfort which another individual can easily tolerate. In IBS this is true for the colon and rectum as well as the small intestine. So their management must be directed to all these measures we have talked about above in the treatment of the IBS.

Much has been written and advertised about some substances that are supposed to reduce gas symptoms; they are prescribed alone as simethicone (Mylicon is one well known) or in combination with antacids. They are supposed to break up large collections of bubbles of gas and thus relieve symptoms. How effective they are is really not known, but they are worth a trial, and are certainly harmless. Activated charcoal has quite a vogue, but convincing evidence about its usefulness is scanty.

Obviously, if we move our bowels easily and completely, we will have less undigested food residues available for the intestinal bacteria to feast on, so correction of any tendency toward constipation (discussed in detail in Chapter 4) is clearly in order. But as I have already emphasized, there are limits to amounts of roughage and high-fiber diets individuals raised on low-fiber diets can tolerate.

If foodstuffs are hurried along the intestinal tract by laxatives or emotional stress, then the unabsorbed portion of the foodstuffs will enter the colon to be acted upon by the colonic bacteria. So these factors require attention.

If you are one of those numerous individuals who suffers from lactose intolerance, the inability to digest lactose (the sugar of milk), then this too will add further unabsorbed carbohydrates (sugars) to the diet of your colonic bacterial inhabitants and so release more gas.

It might be useful at this point to list the so-called gaseous vegetables. They include navy beans, soybeans, lima beans, onions, broccoli, cabbage, cauliflower, brussels sprouts, kohlrabi, radishes, cucumbers, and celery. Flatulence is increased by apple, grape, and prune juice, raisins and bananas, but curiously not by orange juice or apricot nectar.

12

Sexually Transmitted Bowel Diseases (STBD)

A book devoted to information for the general public regarding bowel disorders would, in my opinion, be deficient if even a brief discussion of the subject of sexually transmitted bowel diseases (STBD) were omitted. I should emphasize that this section is not centered around the widely popularized and disturbing disease of the *acquired immune deficiency syndrome* (AIDS). The increased sexual freedom of the last decades, however, has led to an increase in the usual STBDs and has been associated with the appearance of AIDS.

Among homosexual men and some heterosexual couples, the rectum is a sexual organ, and this allows for the local transmission of a large number of viruses, bacteria, and parasites. Breaks in the fragile lining of the rectum permit the transfer of an infection by such organisms. The wider sexual contact involving rectum, mouth, and hands allows also for the transmission of organisms that normally live in the intestinal tract—*Shigella* and *Salmonella,* for example, which are more frequently derived from eating and drinking infected food or water, and such viruses as hepatitis A and hepatitis B and cytomegalovirus (CMV as it is usually abbreviated).

Gonorrhea and *syphilis* have long been known to occur in the rectum. Before the recent explosion of AIDS, infection with the *herpesvirus* was the most widely known and feared disorder. In the lower bowel, herpesvirus (herpes simplex virus, type 2) can cause a proctitis and mimics the nonspecific proctitis discussed in Chapter 3. In addition to the local rectal symptoms, this may also present some wider ones such as pain on urination, and pain in nerves spreading out from the rectal area to the buttocks. The acute symptoms respond to the antiviral agent acyclovir, but unfortunately this medicine does not do much to prevent recurrences.

The commonest *parasites* that fall into the STBD group are *Giardia lamblia* and *Entamoeba histolytica;* the latter causes amebiasis (discussed in Chapter 4). The former usually causes an upper intestinal disturbance with nausea and diarrhea as the main symptoms.

Another group of disorders falling into this group of diseases are the large viruses of the *Chlamydia* family. These can cause much trouble in the rectum and even beyond with inflammation and abscesses, fistulas, and scarring with strictures, which at first glance and even under longer observation, resemble Crohn's disease (Chapter 3). Recently an association between one of this group, *Chlamydia trachomatis* and Crohn's has been sought intensively, but has not been found. The inflammation caused by this organism responds to treatment with the antibiotic oxytetracycline.

Among both doctors and laypeople, the term *gay bowel syndrome* has been applied to this group of disorders, but it does not describe a specific disease syndrome (which is a constellation of symptoms); it refers rather to a list of conditions. What makes the problem difficult is that STBD may mimic some of the other bowel disorders discussed in this volume, and often the causes may be several organisms present at the same time. Although in some individuals the infections or infestations show no symptoms, most have rectal pain, rectal burning, disturbance in bowel movements (either an increased number of looseness, or in some, painful defecation, which leads to constipation) plus the passage of mucus and even rectal bleeding.

Given this large group of infectious diseases of the colon and rectum, especially their resemblance to the important nonspecific inflammation (ulcerative colitis and Crohn's disease), and the importance of distinguishing them carefully in order to start the appropriate drug treatments, it will become clear to you why today's treating physician must determine the sexual preferences of the patient. He or she must consider the anus and rectum as a sexual organ, and remember that several infections are frequently present together. This means that careful studies of blood, biopsy of tissues, and repeated examinations of stools must be done to find the offending agent or agents (Table 12.1).

To make the situation even more complicated, patients whose immune systems have been rendered incompetent or suppressed by the human T-lymphotropic virus (HTLVIII) (believed responsible for the AIDS syndrome), or whose immune defenses have been destroyed or impaired by cancer or anticancer drugs, can now fall prey to a number of infections which ordinarily they could easily withstand. The list grows larger each day as researchers in the field turn them up: herpes simplex virus, herpes zoster, which causes

TABLE 12.1 Sexually Transmissible Diseases

Intestinal Infections	Nonintestinal Infections
Parasites	*Classical venereal diseases*
Amebiasis, giardiasis	Syphilis
Pinworms, cysticercosis,	gonorrhea
strongyloidiasis	*Others*
Viruses	Genital herpes
Hepatitis A and B	trichomoniasis
CMV	*Chlamydia*
Bacteria	
Shigellosis	
salmonellosis	

shingles, cytomegalic virus, the parasite *Cryptosporidum,* which was thought never to cause human disease. These "opportunistic infections," as they are now called, include *fungi* of the *Candida* family, which cause the infection in the mouth and throat called *thrush,* formerly found only in malnourished babies or in patients receiving antibiotics, as well as a bacterium that resembles the one causing tuberculosis but is an atypical form that can cause inflammation in the colon indistinguishable from ulcerative colitis. Biopsies of the colon or rectal lining need to be specially stained to find this *Mycobacteria (avium-intracellulare)* to treat it as needed.

It is important to remember, however, despite the grim tone of this account, that these bowel problems are really quite rare in the general population, and rightly deserve only a small amount of space in a volume such as this.

13

The Abdominal Pain
Without a Name

There are, unfortunately, instances in which someone complains of a chronic abdominal pain for which no cause is found, even after a prolonged serious search is made. Not only the pain, but the fact that our doctors cannot give us a diagnostic label for the cause, increases our anxiety. Fortunately, these cases are uncommon, but not so rare as to be unusual. Sometimes the cause of the original problem clears up but the pain persists. Other times, all disease has been removed by abdominal surgery, yet pain persists. It is like the pain of a "phantom limb": The limb is gone but the pain persists. Sufferers go from doctor to doctor and submit to endless repetition of uninformative tests seeking relief. The pain without a name is no joke.

Whatever the reason, the former ulcer, gallbladder, pancreas, intestinal, or colonic problem has now become a "pain problem." Because of this, much recent research has focused on pain, and centers for the study and treatment of chronic pain have been founded. These pain clinics, also called chronic pain centers, aim to treat a condition that often renders the individual dependent on or addicted to painkilling drugs.

New theories of pain physiology and new information about the body's own painkilling chemicals have been utilized in treating the individual with the chronic pain of unknown origin. However, pain clinics insist on the most careful studies, done in great detail, to be sure that subject does not have any organic causes for his or her pain.

You may have read about the *gate control theory of pain*. This theory proposes that certain nerve connections in the spinal cord open or close the "door" to the transmission of pain impulses from the body. The action of the "door" depends on the stimulation of certain nerves with large diameters, which block the transmission of pain sensations to the brain. To take advantage of this phenomenon, the skin is stimulated by electricity, acupuncture, acupressure, massage, or thermal stimulation.

Many pain clinics use *transcutaneous electrical stimulation* for the management of chronic pain. Electrodes are placed near the painful area or over a nerve going to or from the painful area and stimulated. This approach is noninvasive and may give pain relief. These techniques may slowly release the body's own narcotic substances, the endodorphins or the enkephalins, which go to specific areas in the brain, the opiate receptors, near the pain perception center, and block the awareness of pain.

The brain's awareness of pain and the threshold for the awareness may be altered by other techniques, such as behavioral modification, biofeedback, hypnosis, and psychotherapy. These methods are potentially very useful, although exactly how they work is far from clear. For example, the reduction of pain after acupuncture may be due to release of the body's own opiates, the intense sensory stimulation with the twisting needles, or effects on the branches of the nerve themselves.

14

Your Gut Feelings
The Brain–Gut Connection

If philosophy, as someone is reported to have said, is finding better reasons for what one believes on instinct, then psychosomatic medicine is the attempt to prove by science what one feels about the intestine on instinct. This belief that the discomforts and disturbances of the gut arise from disturbances in our feeling and emotions has a long history. We "know" that fear can make our heart beat faster, dilate our pupils, dry our mouths, and loosen our bowels. We knew all about this long before the term *psychosomatic* was coined.

The "solar plexus," the supposed seat of our deeper feelings, was located by the ancients within the abdomen. Not only our grandmothers, but we ourselves know that the workings of our intestinal tract from one end to the other are sensitive to the state of our feelings. The lower intestinal tract (the small intestine and the colon and rectum), which has been the focus of this book, has a limited repertory and thus can react to disturbances in only a few ways. We can have discomfort that varies in intensity from mild to

187

severe pain with intermittent cramps or continuing sustained spasms. Our bowels may refuse to move and empty out our colon (constipation) or move too rapidly, so we have frequent or loose watery stools (diarrhea); or they may react to irritation by pouring out the protective jelly called mucus, or the fragile intestinal lining may bleed.

The basic questions have always been two. How do our feeling states and emotions work their effect on the intestinal tract? Second, can and do these feeling states lead not merely to disturbance (dysfunction) but to disease (organic changes) in the lower bowel?

Until fairly recently, the connection between the emotional centers of the brain and the intestinal tract was believed to be solely by way of the connecting nerve pathways. Some discoveries about the chemistry of the brain have caused a revolution in our thinking about the brain and the gut. It has been long known that the intestine communicates with different parts of itself or its attendant glands (liver, pancreas, gallbladder) by chemical messengers called hormones. These hormones are long chains of amino acids (the building blocks of proteins) known as peptides, which are assembled in specialized cells of the intestine (especially in the stomach and small bowel). The hormones released into the bloodstream signal intestinal muscles to contract, valves to open or close, glands to secrete water, acid, or bicarbonate, specialized cells to pour forth digestive enzymes, and the whole intestine to behave in a smooth, harmonious fashion.

Now, with the revolution in neuroscience, we have learned that these chains of amino acids, the *peptides,* are present in the brain and its far-flung nerves. These chemical messengers are not merely stored in the parts of the nervous system, but are actually manufactured there. With them, the nervous system not only transfers information within itself, but can also signal other parts of the body directly. Interestingly, each gland in the body usually manufactures its own special hormones; only the thyroid makes thyroxine, for example, whereas the ovary makes its own sex hormones. The brain and the gut on the other hand can and do make identical substances, and can thus talk directly to each other. The answers are far from complete, but it is becoming clearer how disturbances in our emotional states, which lead to changes in the chemical activity of the brain, can in turn send disturbing messages to the intestine, and how the intestine in turn can "talk back" to the brain. We are beginning to understand how "brain feelings" can express themselves as gut feelings.

However, there are large gaps in our understanding even of the most studied intestinal problem: the secretion of acid by the stomach. If ulcers of the stomach and duodenum have something to do with stress and tensions, then it would be important to know what emotions do to the stomach's manufacture of acid. Unfortunately, the problem is hard to study; just swallowing a stomach tube to be able to get samples of the acid alters the secretion. Even more puzzling are the different results that various researchers have reported. The most unexpected and disturbing finding is that strong emotions seem to cut down and suppress acid in the stomach.

When it comes to the question of what effects feelings, emotions, and stress have on the function of the lower intestinal tract, the situation is even more obscure. Very little good research has been done on this problem. However, the newer methods of detecting minute amounts of the brain and gut hormones present in the blood offer the very real possibility that we will soon have sound reports on their effects on the lower bowel's actions.

The question of whether repeated disturbances in function due to a person's emotional state can lead to actual diseases of the gut has been a much harder one to answer. At present there is no firm consensus among researchers. For much of this century a group of diseases was considered to be of purely *psychological* origin. These "classic seven" were peptic ulcer, high blood pressure, bronchial asthma, neurodermatitis, overactive thyroid disease (hyperthyroidism), ulcerative colitis, and rheumatoid arthritis, and each was supposed to go with a specific personality type. These "psychosomatic" diseases were believed to bridge the gap between functional disturbances and organic structural disease.

However, increasing experience and study have blurred this simple picture. The idea of specific personality types prone to develop a given disease did not stand up. The link between the psychological functions in the individual's life and the change in their tissues has not been demonstrated. Now emphasis has shifted from the emotional unconscious to the stress of everyday life. Scales have been devised to rate the degree of stress major life events can induce, and investigators then try to correlate an individual's degree of stress with the degree of activity of the disease.

Thus the investigators in this field are not looking at stress for *the* cause of any disease whose origin is unknown, but rather trying to find out how stress influences the course of an illness and to what degree, and especially how it effects the medical or surgical program of treatment the person is following. In part, this shift in emphasis to stress and psychological aspects of illness reflects the widespread feeling that medicine has become too impersonal, too high-technological. We want our physicians to consider "all of us" as a whole rather than as a collection of organs. In part, it reflects the growing conviction that the investigative techniques of the neurosciences will help researchers make progress in putting the mind and the body together. As a result, the role of stress is no longer looked for only in those illnesses whose cause we don't know, but in all chronic illnesses.

What is the current thinking and what do we really know about stress-related factors and those lower abdominal problems we have been discussing throughout this volume? Let us look at the wide range.

At one end of the spectrum are those like the *acute diarrheas*, caused by specific bacteria and viruses, which seem to be very little influenced by psychological components. Yet not everyone exposed to these specific organisms comes down with the illness. Perhaps differences in resistance even to these invaders are due to differences in the state of our immune systems, which protect us against infection and which have been shown to be influenced not only by our nutritional conditions but by our feeling states. Depression seems to lower resistance.

At the other end of the spectrum is the *irritable bowel syndrome,* which most experienced physicians believe has very large emotional and stress-related factors at work in it. As sufferers from the condition, we too feel that this is the case. The most convincing evidence at present is our own observations of the relationship between our feeling states and the distress we experience in our colons; however, this is autobiographic not scientific knowledge. The best evidence from the laboratory is the series of reports of Dr. Thomas Almy, then at Cornell Medical School, who observed the change in lower bowel movements and pressures when unpleasant or painful experiences were discussed with the subject. I am sure we shall see an increasing number of studies of this commonest of all gastrointestinal disorders as soon as better noninvasive electrical and mechanical observations can be made on individuals during the course of daily life. Just as monitors of heart action under similar circumstances have advanced our understanding of dysrhythmias of the cardiovascular system, we will soon know more about electrical dysrhythmias of the bowel. The only psychological state that has been clearly associated with the irritable bowel syndrome has been depression, which certainly needs treatment along with the bowel symptoms.

There are also differences within these groups of illnesses. The two main ones in the *inflammatory bowel disease* group (IBD) seem to be different one from the other. Stress and emotional factors influence *ulcerative colitis* more profoundly then they do *Crohn's disease,* or so it appears at present, yet the sufferers of both see some relation between their disease and their problems. These bald statements are based mainly upon physician's observations of their patients over long periods of time. Although they are not based upon "hard" scientific data, they are not to be disregarded. It is simply that researchers have not yet been able to devise the necessary methods for investigating the problem. It is especially difficult to separate the role of emotions in influencing the course of IBD from the effect that these chronic illnesses, occurring at certain periods in their young sufferers' lives, have upon their emotional states and behavior.

Diverticulosis and *diverticulitis* seem to be more dependent on dietary habits than on the everyday wear and tear of daily life.

Polyps and *cancer* of the intestine are more closely tied to our genetic inheritance and our environment, including dietary factors, than to emotional factors. Yet our immune system, the vigilante devices which protect us against the sporadic wild and malignant cells that turn up from time to time, can be profoundly depressed by feeling states, especially grief and mourning.

So we must conclude for the time being that emotional turmoil and daily stress play a part along with our customary eating habits, the use of alcohol, caffeine, and tobacco, and general lifestyles, including exercise, in how our gut "feels" and its physical condition. The fraction each of these factors plays must be thoughtfully reviewed by both sufferer and physician. In such a careful analysis it may become apparent that for some individuals a consultation with a psychiatrist, psychologist, or psychotherapist is as much in order as the consultations with the gastroenterologist or the radiologist. Although I have not found formal psychoanalysis helpful for my patients, counseling directed at pinpointing the real stresses of the present and ways of handling them has been of considerable use to them.

Many forms of relaxation techniques are available, including reading texts and listening to taped instructions. Physicians now use them in treating high blood pressure before and along with dietary and drug treatments. There is a place for this approach in helping yourself to help your spastic bowel.

Although I cannot entirely agree with Norman Cousins, who in his *Anatomy of an Illness* felt that his own serious immunological illness was cured by laughter and good humor, I certainly can agree that an optimistic mind-set with cheerfulness and the cultivation of fun have tided many patients over the difficult course of their intestinal illnesses.

The term *behavioral modification* covers the whole group of psychological methods of counseling, suggestion, and self-hypnosis, which help individuals to alter and abandon their self-destructive habits of behaving, eating, and dependence on drugs, especially the painkillers, alcohol, and tobacco. This approach, which focuses on altering the present rather than on understanding the past, can be very useful as well.

In the section on the aging gut (Chapter 8) the use of biofeed-back was emphasized in discussing the problem of bowel control. We now know that many actions of the body's organs, formerly thought to be completely automatic and not under our control, can be brought under voluntary control by the techniques of biofeed-back. In a series of demonstrations with audiovisual devices, all of us can be taught to control and lower our blood pressures or slow our heart rate. Similarly, we can learn to lower the pressure in our lower bowels and relax colonic muscles or contractions, as well as contract these muscles. In selected situations, this method can be used to supplement and reinforce the other techniques I have discussed in this chapter to improve our gut feelings.

Suggested Reading

Irritable Bowel Syndrome, edited by N. W. Read. Grune & Stratton, London, 1985. The U.S. edition is published by Grune & Stratton, Inc., Orlando, Florida 32887.

Inflammatory Bowel Disease: A Personal View, H. D. Janowitz. Field, Rich and Associates, Inc., New York, 1985. Distributed by Year Book Medical Publishers, Chicago, Illinois.

Clinical Reactions to Food, edited by M. H. Lesoff. John Wiley, Chichester, London, 1983.

Adverse Reactions to Food. American Academy of Allergy, Committee on Adverse Reactions to Foods. National Institute of Allergy and Infectious Diseases. U.S. Dept. of Health and Human Services. National Institute of Health. NIH Publications, No. 84-2442, Fall 1984.

Burkett, D. P., Walker, A. R. P., and Painter, N. S. *Dietary fiber and disease. Journal of the American Medical Association,* 229:1068–1074, 1974.

Dietary Fiber in Health and Disease, edited by G. V. Vahouny and D. Kritchersky. New York, Plenum, 1982.

Dietary Fibre, Fibre-Depleted Foods and Disease, edited by H. Trowell, D. Burkett, and K. Heston. Academic Press, London, 1985.

Index

Abcess, 138, 140
Abdominal angina, 163
Abdominal epilepsy, 167–68
Abdominal migraine, 167–68
Acid, 5
Acquired immune deficiency syndrome
    (AIDS), 181, 183
Acute diarrhea, 88–89
Acute intermittent porphyria, 167, 176
Acute pancreatitis, 167
Adenoma, 116
Aging gut, 156–64
AIDS, 181, 183
Alcohol
    inflammatory bowel disease, 52
    irritable bowel syndrome, 25–26
    porphyria, 176
Allergies. See Food allergies
Aluminum hydroxide, 173
Amitriptyline (Elavil), 173
Amoeba, 85, 88
Amphojel, 173
Ampicillin, 62
Anatomy of an Illness (Cousins), 192

Anemia, 128–29
Angina, 162–63
Angiodysplasia, 161–62
Angiogram, 109, 163–64
Animal fat. See also Fat
    colon cancer, 114, 127
Antacids, 171, 173
Antibiotic associated diarrhea, 174
Antibiotics
    and absorption, 169–71
    adverse reactions, 174–75
    diverticulitis, 140, 143
    inflammatory bowel disease, 62
Anticholinergics, 28
Anticoagulants, 175
Antidepressants
    constipation effect, 173
    irritable bowel syndrome, 29
Antigen-antibody complexes, 46
Antihistamines, 155
Antiinflammatory medicine, 59–63
Antispasmodics, 28
Anus, 7
Appendix, 13

Arthritis, 46
Ascending colon, 6
Aspirin, 175
Atropine, 28
Autonomic nervous system, 30–31
Azathioprine (Imuran), 63, 74
Azulfadine. *See* Sulfasalazine

Bacillus cereus, 82
Bacteria
    and aging, 157
    in human colon, 8
Bactrim, 81, 85, 87
Barbiturates, 176
Barium enema
    in diverticulitis, 139
    inflammatory bowel disease, 48–49
    and irritable bowel syndrome, 20–23
Behavioral modification, 192
Belladonna, 28
Bentyl, 28
Bile acid, 127–28
Biofeedback, 193
    fecal incontinence, 160–61
    irritable bowel syndrome, 3
Biopsy, 49
Bismuth subsalicylate (Pepto-Bismol), 80, 85, 172
Bladder, 141–42
Bleeding. *See also* Rectal bleeding
    and aging, 161–62
    colon cancer sign, 128–29
Bowel pattern, 129
Bran, in constipation, 103
Bread, fiber content, 100
Burkett, D.P., 136

Caffeine
    inflammatory bowel disease, 52
    irritable bowel syndrome, 25
Calcium absorption, 157
Calcium carbonate, 173
Calcium-channel blockers, 176
Calcium lactate, 173
Calcium-rich foods, 126
Calcium supplements
    adverse reactions, 172–73
    colon cancer, 115
    inflammatory bowel disease, 57
Campylobacter, 38, 80–82, 85, 87
Cancer. *See* Colon cancer

Candida family, 184
Carbon dioxide, 178–79
Carcinoembryonic antigen test (CEA test), 125
Cascara, 174
CEA test, 125
Cecal diverticulitis, 144
Cecum, 6
Cereals, fiber content, 100
Chemotherapy, 130
Childbirth, 74
Chinese restaurant syndrome, 149
Chlamydia family, 182
Cholesterol, 127
Chronic diarrhea, 89–94
Cigarette smoking. *See* Smoking
Cimetidine (Tagamet), 173
Circular intestinal muscles, 11
Claustridia, 87, 175
Clindamycin, 62
Clostridium botulinum, 82
Codeine, 63–64
Coeliac disease, 94
Colace, 103
Colan (verapamil), 176
Colitis. *See* Ulcerative colitis
Colon
    diagram, 6
    digestive process, 6, 36
    pain location, 12–13
Colon cancer, 112–32
    and aging, 158–59
    causes, 113–15
    definition, 112
    diagnosis, 129–30
    diet, 114–15
    and diverticular disease, 143
    emotional factors, 192
    incidence, 113
    and inflammatory bowel diseases, 70–71
    prevention, 127
    prognosis, 130
    symptoms, 128–29
    treatment, 130–32
Colonoscopy, 49, 71, 119–20
Colostomy, 68–69, 131, 140–41
Conjunctivitis, 45
Constipation, 78–111
    causes, 98
    definition, 78–94

and diabetes, 166
and fiber, 98–102
irritable bowel syndrome, 18
and lifestyle, 105
medicines, 28
psychology, 96
tests for, 97
Continent ileostomy, 69
Contraceptive pills, 175
"Core diet," 154–55
Cortisone drugs. *See* Steroids
Cotton top marmoset, 42
Coumadin, 175
Counseling, 33–34
Cousins, Norman, 192
Cow's milk, 152
Cramps
  medicines, 28, 63
  muscle contraction, 10
Crohn's disease, 35–77
  and cancer, 72
  diet, 53–58, 152
  and diverticula, 142
  extraintestinal manifestations, 45–46
  and maturation, 44
  medications, 58–64, 75–77
  psychology, 66, 191
  surgery, 68–70
  symptoms, 43–44
  treatment results, 67
  versus ulcerative colitis, 36–33
Cromolyn, 155
Cryptosporidum, 184
Cutaneous nerves, 8–9

Dairy products. *See also* Milk
  inflammatory bowel disease, 54
Depression, 24, 33–34, 191
Dermatitis herpetiformis, 150
Descending colon, 6
Diabetes, 166
Diarrhea, 78–111
  and aging, 159
  definition, 78
  and diabetes, 166
  irritable bowel syndrome, 18
  medicines, 28, 63–64
  treatment, 80–81
Diet
  colon cancer, 114

Crohn's disease, 152
inflammatory bowel disease, 53–58
irritable bowel syndrome, 26–28
Diet, Nutrition and Cancer (National
  Academy Press), 115
Dietary fiber. *See* Fiber
Dilantin (Phenytoin), 170–71
Diphenoxylate (Lomotil), 28, 63, 80, 86,
  166
Diuretics
  adverse reactions, 174, 176
  secretory diarrhea, 91
Diverticula, 133–45, 159
Diverticulitis, 133–45
  and aging, 159
  and cancer, 143
  characteristics, 138–39
  diagnosis, 139
  and perforation, 141–42
  prognosis, 142–43
  treatment, 139–41
Diverticulosis, 133–45
Donnatal, 28, 63
Doxycycline (Vibramycin), 85
Drugs, 169–76
Duhring's disease, 150
Duke's stages, 130
Duodenum, 5, 36
Dysplasia, 72

E. coli, 80–82, 85, 88
Elavil (amitriptyline), 173
Elemental diet, 154
Elimination diets, 147–48, 153–54
Emotions, 24, 187–93
Endocrine glands, 165
Enemas. *See also* Barium enema
  and constipation, 104
Entamoeba hystolytica, 87, 90, 182
Environmental factors, 113–14
Eosinophilic gastroenteritis, 152
Erythema nodosum, 46
Erythromycin, 81
Esophagus, 4–5
Estrogen, 175
Ex-Lax, 174
Exercise, 29–30, 64–65
External rectal sphincter
  digestive process, 7
  and incontinence, 160–61

Familial polyposis, 113, 125–57
Fat
    colon cancer, 114, 127
    inflammatory bowel disease, 54
    malabsorption syndromes, 93
Fecal incontinence, 159–61, 166
Fertility, 75
Fiber, 109–11
    and bowel symptoms, 23, 26–27
    colon cancer, 114–15, 127
    and constipation, 98–102
    in diet, table, 100–2
    and diverticula, 136, 142, 144–45
    inflammatory bowel disease, 56
    and prevention, 110
Fiber Med, 102
Riber Rich, 102
Fistulas
    Crohn's disease, 40
    diverticulitis, 141–42
Flagyl. *See* Metronidazole
Fleets enema, 48
Flexible colonoscope, 21–22
Flexible endoscope, 48
Flexible sigmoidoscope, 21, 49
Flexical, 154
Fluid, and polyps, 120–21
Fluid intake, 104–5
Folic acid, 57, 170
Food allergies, 146–55
    diagnosis, 147–48, 153–55
    diets, 153–55
    drug treatment, 155
    irritable bowel syndrome, 27
    symptoms, 147, 150
Food idiosyncracy, 148
Food intolerance, 148–49
    definition, 148–49
    diarrhea, 91
    inflammatory bowel disease, 54
    irritable bowel syndrome, 24, 26–28
Food poisoning, 81–82
Food supplements, 56–58
Fruit, fiber content, 100
Functional disturbances, 16–17

Gallbladder
    malabsorption syndromes, 93
    pain location, 11–12
Garamycin, 62
Gas, 177–80

Gastric-colic reflex diarrhea, 89
Gastroenterologists, 47
Gate control pain theory, 186
Gay bowel syndrome, 182
General practitioners, 47
Giardia lamblia, 85, 87, 90, 182
Gluten, 27
Gluten enteropathy, 150–51
Gonorrhea, 182
Granulomas, 40

Hair analysis, 147
Heart disease, 176
Hemoccult test, 122–24
Hemoglobin, 123–24
HemoQuant, 123–24
Herpesvirus, 182
High-fiber diet
    bowel symptoms, 23, 26
    colon cancer, 114
    and constipation, 98–102
    and diverticula, 144–45
    inflammatory bowel disease, 56
High-fiber/low-carbohydrate diet, 152
High-protein diet, 54
High-sugar/low-fiber diet, 152
Hirschsprung's disease, 95, 105–6
Hormones, 188
Hyperthyroidism, 165
Hypothyroidism, 166

Ileostomy, 68–69
Ileum, 5, 36
Immunosuppressant drugs, 62–63
Imodium, 28, 80, 86, 89, 166
Imuran (azathioprine), 63, 74
Incontinence, 159–61, 166
Inderal, 176
Inflammatory bowel disease, 35–77
    and aging, 158
    and cancer, 70–72
    and diet, 53–58
    and diverticula, 142
    extraintestinal manifestations, 45–46
    versus irritable bowel syndrome, 16
    and lifestyle, 64–65
    medications, 58–64
    and pregnancy, 73
    psychology, 65–66, 191

surgery, 68–70
tests and examination, 48–49
treatment results, 67–68
Inflammatory diseases, definition, 38
Inflammatory polyps, 117
Internal sphincters
digestive process, 7
and incontinence, 160–61
Intestinal gas, 177–80
Intestinal obstruction, 45
Intestinal resection, 68–69
"Intestinal virus," 79, 81
Iron, 57
Iron pills, 172
Irritable bowel syndrome, 14–34
common patient complaints, 17–18
diagnosis, 18–22
and diverticula, 144–45
versus inflammatory bowel diseases,
16
and intestinal gas, 179
and lifestyle, 32–33
psychology, 24, 33–34, 190–91
relaxation techniques, 30–32
stress, 29–30
treatment, 22–25, 28–29
Ischemic colitis, 164, 175

Jejunum, 5, 36
Jews, 40–41

Kaopectate, 86, 89
Kock pouch, 69

LactAid, 26, 55, 149
Lactase, 149
Lactose, 149
Lactose intolerance, 149
characteristics, 149
diarrhea, 91
inflammatory bowel disease, 54–55
intestinal gas, 180
irritable bowel syndrome, 24, 26
Lactose tolerance test, 26, 55
Laxatives, 104, 174
Levitt, Michael, 177
Librax, 28, 63
Listeria monocytogenes, 88
Liver
and malabsorption syndromes, 93
pain location, 11

Lomotil, 28, 63, 80, 86, 89, 166
Longitudinal intestinal muscles, 11
Loperamide (Imodium), 28, 63, 80,
86, 166
Lower intestinal tract, 3–13
Lubricants, 103–4

Maalox, 173
Malabsorption syndromes, 89–94
Male fertility, 75
Malnutrition, 92
Margarine, 153–54
Masked hyperthyroidism, 165–66
Maturation, and Crohn's disease, 44
Meat, fiber content, 101
Medicines, 169–76
Megacolon, 106
Melanosis coli, 97
6-Mercaptopurine, 63, 74
Metamucil, 28, 145
Metronidazole
and alcohol, 52
Crohn's disease, 62
Milk
fiber content, 101
inflammatory bowel disease, 54–55,
152
irritable bowel syndrome, 26
Milk of magnesia, 173
Minerals, 56–58
Monosodium glutamate, 149
Motility studies, 97
Mucosa, and polyps, 116
Mucus, and polyps, 120
Multivitamins, 27–28, 57
Muscle contractions
irritable bowel syndrome, 24
sensations, 10
Mylicon, 179

Nalcrom, 155
Nicotine, 25
Nursing mothers, 74
Nutrition, Crohn's disease, 53

Oncogenes, 113
Ostomy, 68–69

Pain, 185–86
colon cancer sign, 128–29

Pain, continued
  in intestine, origin, 8–10
  location, 11–13
  relaxation techniques, 30–31
  treatment, 186
Pancreas
  malabsorption syndromes, 93–94
  pain location, 12
"Pancreatic cholera," 91
Pancreatitis, 167, 174
Parasites, 89–90
  sexually transmitted diseases, 182
  tests for, 90
  traveler's diarrhea, 85
Parathyroid glands, 166–67
Parotid salivary gland, 4
Pathibamate, 63
Pelvic pouch, 69
Peppermint oil, 28
Pepsin, 5
Peptides, 188
Pepto-Bismol, 80, 85, 172
Perforation, 141–42
Personality types, 189–90
Phenytoin (Dilantin), 170–71
Physical exercise, 29–30
"Picket-fence" diverticula, 136–37
Polyps, 112–32
  and aging, 159
  prevention, 121–25
  removal, 124
  symptoms, 120–21
  types of, 116–18
Porphyrin, 167, 176
Prediverticular phase, 136–37
Pregnancy, 73–74
Procardia, 176
Proctitis, 36, 42–43
Proctoscopy, 48
Propranolol, 176
Protein, 54
Pseudomembranous colitis, 175
"Pseudo obstructions," 96, 106–7
Pseudopolyps, 118–20
Psychoanalysis, 66
Psychology, 189–90
Psychosomatic medicine, 187–93
Psychotherapy
  inflammatory bowel diseases, 66
  irritable bowel syndrome, 33–34

Psyllium seeds, 98, 103
Purinethol, 63
Pyoderma gangrenosum, 46

Quinidine, 176

Radiating pain, 11
Radiation
  colon cancer, 130
  rectal cancer, 131
Radioallergosorbent tests, 147
Ranitidine (Zantac), 173
Raynaud's phenomenon, 96
Rectal bleeding, 78, 107–9. *See also*
  Hemoccult test
  and aging, 161–62
  colon cancer, 128–29
  Crohn's disease, 45
  definition, 78
  diverticulitis, 141
  importance, 47
  investigation of, 107–9
  irritable bowel syndrome, 17–18
Rectal cancer, 131
Rectosigmoid colon, 6
Rectum, 7
Referred pain, 9
Regional iletis, 38
Relaxation techniques, 30–31, 192
Resection of the intestine, 68–69,
  140–44
Rice, fiber content, 101
Rigid sigmoidoscope, 20, 48–49
Roughage. *See also* Fiber
  inflammatory bowel disease, 56
  irritable bowel syndrome, 27

Salads, 27
Salazopyrine, 75, 170
Salivary glands, 4–5
Salmonella, 38, 80–82, 85, 181
Schuster, Marvin, 160
Secretory diarrhea, 89–91
"Segmental" colitis, 50
Selenium, 58
Senna, 99
Senokot, 99
Sensations, intestines, 8–10
Septra, 81, 85, 87

"Sessile" polyps, 116, 119, 124–25
Sexually transmitted bowel diseases, 181–84
Shigella, 38, 80–81, 85, 182
Sigmoid colitis, 36
Sigmoid colon
    diverticulosis, 136, 140, 143–44
    irritable bowel syndrome, 19
    pain location, 13
Sigmoid colostomies, 131
Sigmoid resection, 143–44
Sigmoidoscopy
    constipation, 97
    inflammatory bowel disease, 48–49
    irritable bowel syndrome, 19–20
    recent developments, 20
Silent diverticula, 144
Simethicone, 179–80
Skin conditions, 46
Skin tests, 147
Slow viruses, 42
Small intestine
    gastrointestinal tract, 5, 36–37
    and malabsorption syndromes, 94
    pain location, 12–13
Smoking
    colon cancer, 115
    inflammatory bowel disease, 51–52
    irritable bowel syndrome, 25
Sodium cromoglycate, 155
Sodium dioctyl sulfate, 103
Somatic nerves, 8–9
Sorbitol, 173–74
Spasms, 10
Spastic colon, 18. *See also* Irritable bowel syndrome
Sperm count, 75
Sphincter muscles
    digestive process, 7
    and incontinence, 160–61
Sports, 64
Sprue, 150–51
Stalk polyps, 116–18, 124
Staphylococci, 82, 88
Steroids
    inflammatory bowel disease, 60–61
    side effects, 60–61
Stomach
    and malabsorption syndromes, 93
    pain location, 12

Stool examination
    inflammatory bowel disease, 48
    polyps, 121–24
Stress
    exercise effects, 29–30
    irritable bowel syndrome, 24, 29–30
    and psychosomatics, 189–92
Structural disturbances, 16–17
Sublingual salivary gland, 4
Submaxillary gland, 4
Sulfa drugs, 176
Sulfasalazine
    inflammatory bowel disease, 59–60, 67
    side effects, 59
Suppositories, 104
Surveillance, 71–72
Syphilis, 182

Tagamet (cimetidine), 173
Tetracyclines, 62, 169, 171
Thyroid gland, 165–66
Tincture of belladonna, 28
Tobacco, 25
Total Parenteral Nutrition, 58
"Toxic dilation of the colon," 43
"Trace elements," 57–58
Transcendental meditation, 31
Transcutaneous electrical stimulation, 186
Transit time, 97
Transverse colon, 6
Traveler's diarrhea, 82–87
Tricyclic antidepressants, 173
Trimethoprim/sulfamethoxazole, 81, 85–86
True polyps, 116
True visceral pain, 9
"Tubular polyps," 116
Tums, 173

Ulcerative colitis, 35–77
    and cancer, 70–72
    versus Crohn's disease, 36–38
    diet, 53–58
    and diverticula, 142
    extraintestinal manifestations, 45–46
    medications, 58–64
    psychology, 65–66, 191

Ulcerative colitis, continued
  surgery, 68–70
  symptoms, 42–43
  treatment, 50–64, 67
Universal ulcerative colitis
  definition, 36
  symptoms, 43

Vegetables
  colon cancer, 114–15
  fiber content, 101–2
Verapamil (Colan), 176
Vibramycin, 85
Vibrio cholerae, 82
Villous adenoma, 120–21
"Villous polyps," 116

Visceral nerve sets, 8–9
Vitamin B$_{12}$, 57, 170–71
Vitamin C, 57
Vitamin D, 157
Vitamin supplements, 27–28, 56–58
Vivonex, 154

Weaning, 152
Wheat intolerance, 150–51

Yersinia, 80
Yoga, 31
Yogurt, 26

Zantac (ranitidine), 173
Zinc, 57–58